FETAL ALCOHOL SYNDROME

Diagnosis, Epidemiology, Prevention, and Treatment

Kathleen Stratton, Cynthia Howe, and Frederick Battaglia, *Editors*

Committee to Study Fetal Alcohol Syndrome

Division of Biobehavioral Sciences
and Mental Disorders

INSTITUTE OF MEDICINE

NATIONAL ACADEMY PRESS
Washington, D.C.   1996

NATIONAL ACADEMY PRESS • 2101 Constitution Ave., N.W. • Washington, D.C. 20418

NOTICE: The project that is the subject of this report was approved by the Governing Board of the National Research Council, whose members are drawn from the councils of the National Academy of Sciences, the National Academy of Engineering, and the Institute of Medicine. The members of the committee responsible for the report were chosen for their special competencies and with regard for appropriate balance.

This report has been reviewed by a group other than the authors according to procedures approved by a Report Review Committee consisting of members of the National Academy of Sciences, the National Academy of Engineering, and the Institute of Medicine.

The Institute of Medicine was chartered in 1970 by the National Academy of Sciences to enlist distinguished members of the appropriate professions in the examination of policy matters pertaining to the health of the public. In this the Institute acts under the Academy's 1863 congressional charter responsibility to be an adviser to the federal government and, upon its own initiative, to identify issues of medical care, research, and education. Dr. Kenneth I. Shine is President of the Institute of Medicine.

The project was supported by funds from the National Institute on Alcohol Abuse and Alcoholism (contract no. NO1-AA-4-1002).

The serpent has been a symbol of long life, healing, and knowledge among almost all cultures and religions since the beginning of recorded history. The image adopted as a logotype by the Institute of Medicine is based on a relief carving from ancient Greece, now held by the Staatlichemuseen in Berlin.

COMMITTEE TO STUDY FETAL ALCOHOL SYNDROME

Frederick C. Battaglia,* Chair, Professor of Pediatrics, University of Colorado Health Sciences Center, Denver, CO

Hoover Adger, Associate Professor, General Pediatrics/Adolescent Medicine, Johns Hopkins School of Medicine, Baltimore, MD

Nancy C. Andreasen,* Professor of Psychiatry, Mental Health Clinical Research Center, The University of Iowa, Iowa City, IA

Kathleen M. Carroll, Assistant Professor of Psychiatry, Director of Psychotherapy Substance Abuse Center, Yale University School of Medicine, New Haven, CT

Sterling K. Clarren, Professor of Pediatrics, Division of Congenital Defects, Children's Hospital and Medical Center, University of Washington, Seattle, WA

Claire D. Coles, Associate Professor, Department of Psychiatry/Pediatrics, Emory University School of Medicine, Atlanta, GA

Henry W. Foster, Jr.,* Professor, Obstetrics and Gynecology, Meharry Medical College, Nashville, TN

Donald E. Hutchings, Research Scientist, Department of Psychobiology, New York State Psychiatric Institute, New York, NY

Philip A. May, Professor of Sociology and Psychiatry, and Director, Center on Alcoholism, Substance Abuse and Addictions, University of New Mexico, Albuquerque, NM

Bennett A. Shaywitz, Professor of Pediatrics, Neurology and Child Study Center, Yale University School of Medicine, New Haven, CT

Robert J. Sokol, Dean, School of Medicine, Professor, Obstetrics and Gynecology, Wayne State University, Detroit, MI

R. Dale Walker, Professor, Department of Psychiatry and Behavioral Sciences, University of Washington, VA Medical Center, Seattle, WA

Joanne Weinberg, Professor of Anatomy, University of British Columbia, Vancouver, BC, Canada

Sharon C. Wilsnack, Chester Fritz Distinguished Professor, Department of Neuroscience, University of North Dakota School of Medicine, Grand Forks, ND

---

* Member, Institute of Medicine

iii

Project Staff

Kathleen R. Stratton, Project Director
Cynthia J. Howe, Program Officer
Dorothy R. Majewski, Project Assistant
Shanta Henderson, Intern
Jamaine Tinker, Financial Associate
Constance M. Pechura, Director, Division of Biobehavioral Sciences and
    Mental Disorders
Michael A. Stoto, Director, Division of Health Promotion and Disease
    Prevention

Preface

The last 20 years have brought home to most Americans the profound impact of substance abuse on individuals, their families, and society. Most extended families have had some experience with this problem.

We are only recently becoming more aware of the terrible effects of substance abuse on pregnant women and their unborn children. Of all current substance abuse, alcohol is the most serious problem by far, whether judged by its frequency or by its capacity to injure the fetus. In its most obvious form, it leads to a constellation of findings in the infant that are referred to as the fetal alcohol syndrome (FAS).

Because of concerns about the magnitude of the problem, the U.S Congress mandated this study, under the auspices of the Institute of Medicine (IOM) of the National Academy of Sciences. From the outset, the committee was aware of treading on new ground in addressing alcohol abuse during pregnancy since the approach used in this study might serve as a paradigm for other studies of substance abuse in pregnancy. What are the unique characteristics of alcohol abuse in pregnancy that make it such a challenge for medicine and for society in general?

First, this is not a disease that affects only the child with FAS; it involves both the mother and her baby. FAS is a classic example of a family problem. A mother who abuses alcohol needs and deserves treatment for this problem, not only during pregnancy but afterward. If she continues to be alcohol-dependent she may very well die from the disease in a few years and, in the interim, have additional affected pregnancies. Alcohol abuse affects her ability to care properly for her children throughout childhood. The affected child needs continued medical care aimed at minimizing any of the developmental handicaps imposed by FAS. As with many birth defects, optimal care requires coordinated effort from many groups, including providers of health care, social services, and schools.

Secondly, as with many risk factors for a fetus, whether influenced by maternal behavior (e.g., infection with sexually transmitted diseases) or not (e.g., inborn errors of metabolism), if the mother does not receive treatment the effects can be amplified by recurrence, that is by births to that mother of additional affected children, or by the children—when they reach reproductive age—bearing affected infants of their own.

Given these effects of alcohol abuse during pregnancy, the committee addressed the issue of updating the diagnostic criteria that should be used for FAS. We were concerned that, without well-defined criteria, any developmental delay or behavioral abnormality in children whose mothers had any level of alcohol intake might lead to inappropriate labeling with the FAS diagnosis. The criteria recommended are as close as possible to those commonly used by workers in this field and, at the same time, follow the guidelines generally used for setting diagnostic criteria in other areas of medicine.

A consideration of diagnostic criteria brought out the fact that many infants with FAS are not being diagnosed at birth, either because they cannot be or because professionals do not have the tools and training to do so. Pattern recognition is part of the diagnostic criteria in a disease of dysmorphogenesis. In this case it involves recognition of the pattern of facial abnormalities and of the neurobehavioral and developmental characteristics associated with FAS. Who is to be trained for diagnosis in the newborn period, or at any time in childhood? This is an important issue when one considers surveillance approaches that might be applicable on a public health basis. The committee was impressed that this area needs some focused clinical research before widespread surveillance approaches can be recommended. Such research and field testing is considered an urgent priority.

Also relevant to both diagnosis and prevention is the issue of whether there are problems of development or behavior from *any* alcohol intake, no matter how low, during pregnancy. Since this is not yet known, the committee focused on the constellation of infant problems for which good evidence exists of a relationship with maternal abuse of alcohol.

There have been excellent reviews of animal studies relating to FAS. For this reason, the report does not include a detailed review of this topic. Animal models have been established, and studies at the levels of integrative physiology and cell biology have contributed substantially to our understanding of some aspects of the disease. The report attempts to place these basic studies in context in terms of their contribution to our understanding of pathogenesis and prevention. For example, basic research contributed to our understanding of FAS by firmly establishing alcohol as a teratogen. It was also important in highlighting those organ systems likely to be most affected during in utero development. In terms of developmental timing, basic research established the important concept that alcohol can injure the fetus, particularly the central nervous system, not only during embryogenesis, but also later in pregnancy. It was clear to the committee that there are many areas in which additional basic research could make substantial contributions to our understanding of the relationship of dosage, developmental timing, genetic susceptibility, gender differences, and differences in tolerance imposed by the endocrine changes of pregnancy. Such research could contribute by pointing toward additional therapeutic approaches that might be used during pregnancy.

The sections on prevention and treatment once again emphasize that two patients must be considered. Treatment of alcohol abuse and dependence in a pregnant woman is also prevention of FAS in her fetus. The committee wrestled with the difficulty that universal prevention methods appear to have an impact on women with low or moderate alcohol intake but no impact on women who abuse alcohol. Yet, it is this latter group that produces infants with FAS and related problems. Thus, targeting specific prevention and treatment approaches to this latter group is vital if we are to reduce the incidence of FAS. Unfortunately, currently there is little evidence of successful approaches. Too often, we have assumed that whatever works in men who abuse alcohol will work in women who abuse alcohol. This is another area in which clinical research, with strong evaluation components, needs to be implemented.

Treatment of the child begins whenever FAS (or a related disorder) is recognized. The later this recognition occurs in development, the less success treatment protocols will have. For this reason, training medical staff and other gatekeepers in pattern recognition and appropriate history taking in pregnancy is of paramount importance. As with many birth defects, there is a tendency to assume that the damage is done by the time the infant is born. However, this report brings out the lack of knowledge about how much subsequent developmental difficulty is due to actual organic injury at birth, how much is due to the chaotic environment in which most of these children are raised, and how much could be ameliorated by appropriate postnatal intervention and treatment. Such children should not be "discarded" by society and if, as a society, we are sincere in this belief, then the same multidisciplinary approach to their treatment and schooling should be applied as has been used for other birth defects, including joint planning and communication between medical and social services on the one hand and school systems on the other. Stability of the family environment in which the child is reared is necessary for all children, but is often not available to these children. Furthermore, even when these children are raised in stable foster or adoptive homes, appropriate treatment and schooling are often not available.

It is evident throughout the report that fetal alcohol syndrome tests our ability to provide integrated services that cut across medical disciplines to the mother and child. It also presents major challenges to integrating school and support services for these children. The treatment section of the report emphasizes that, where it is uncertain whether developmental and behavioral character-istics are associated with permanent organic injury, children should be given the benefit of the doubt and have access to treatment measures that may substantially improve their outcome. This has been true, over and over again, for other birth defects, and there is no evidence that suggests it will not prove true for FAS.

I would like to acknowledge the diligence of the committee members and thank them for their efforts. Each contributed in a unique way, bringing both area-specific expertise and a broader perspective to the problem. I enjoyed our challenging discussions. I would also like to thank the IOM staff: Kathleen Stratton for her guidance and coordination of committee activities and her pa-tience at seeing this activity through, Constance Pechura for her perspective and help in putting our ideas into words, Dorothy Majewski for arranging our meet-ings and transcribing our scribbled edits, and Cynthia Howe for doing whatever needed to be done and her attention to detail.

Frederick C. Battaglia, M.D.
Chair
Committee to Study Fetal Alcohol Syndrome

Acknowledgments

The committee wishes to acknowledge the dedication and hard work of the following staff members of the National Research Council and the Institute of Medicine in the completion of this project: Laura Baird, Rhashida Beynum, Claudia Carl, Moeen Darwiesh, Michael Edington, Melvin Hairston, Kathi Hand, Carrie Ingalls, Sandra McDermin, Francesca Moghari, Carolyn Peters, Florence Poillon, Barbara Kline Pope, Terri Scanlan, Mary Lee Schneiders, Sally Stanfield, Carlton Stewart, Nancy Stoltzfus, Donna Thompson, Jamaine Tinker, and Sue Wyatt.

The committee also wishes to express its gratitude to the following individuals who have assisted in various ways: Ernest Abel, Mary Applegate, Susan Astley, Thomas Babor, Marvin Bailey, Nancy Day, Peter Delaney, Edward Dembowski, Herman Diesenhaus, Thomas Donaldson, Grace Egeland, Robert Fineman, Louise Floyd, Laurie Foudin, Freda Giblin, Rebecca Goodemoot, Paula Hallberg, John Hannigan, Michelle Herron, Vicki Hild, Charlene Hill-Hamilton, Joseph Hollowell, Gail Houle, Jan Howard, Matthew Howard, Richard Johnston, Michael Katz, Michelle Kiely, Michael Kramer, Valborg Kvigne, Dow Lambert, Jane Lockmuller, Steven Long, Susan Lorenzo, Spero Manson, Ellen Marks, John Middaugh, April Montgomery, Barbara Morse, Patti Munter, Gail Shur, Ann Umemoto, Kay VanderVan, Patricia Silk Walker, Kenneth Warren, Maureen Weeks, Nancy J. White, Margaret Wilmore.

We have endeavored to recognize the contributions of all who have assisted the committee throughout the course of this project and any omissions were not intentional.

Contents

EXECUTIVE SUMMARY   1

1   INTRODUCTION   17
History, 17
The Federal Responsibility for FAS Research, 21
Congressional Interest, 23
The Committee's Focus and Process, 26
Some Important Definitions, 29

2   ISSUES IN RESEARCH ON FETAL DRUG EFFECTS   33
Principles of Teratology and Developmental Toxicology, 36
Susceptible Stages of Development, 37
Susceptible Species and Genotype, 40
Dose-Response Effects, 41
Intervention and Prevention, 45
A Multifactorial Model, 47

3   VIGNETTES   52
Sally, 53
Ann, 54
Lydia, 55
Mark and James, 56
Peter, 58
Mary, 60
Baby Herbert's Mother, 61

xi

4   DIAGNOSIS AND CLINICAL EVALUATION OF
    FETAL ALCOHOL SYNDROME   63
    Purpose of Medical Diagnoses, 63
    Use of Diagnostic Criteria, 64
    Standards for Evaluating Diagnostic Criteria, 64
    Issues in Deciding on Diagnostic Criteria, 66
    Specific Issues to Be Addressed in Identifying Criteria for
      Fetal Alcohol Syndrome, 67
    Evolution of the Diagnosis of Fetal Alcohol Syndrome, 70
    Longitudinal Perspectives on the FAS Diagnosis, 73
    Diagnostic Categories, 74
    Differential Diagnosis, 79
    Clinical Utility of FAS, ARBD, and ARND Diagnoses, 79
    Recommendations: Diagnostic Criteria, 80

5   EPIDEMIOLOGY AND SURVEILLANCE OF
    FETAL ALCOHOL SYNDROME   82
    Incidence and Prevalence of FAS, ARBD, ARND, 82
    Surveillance Methods for Fetal Alcohol Syndrome, 91
    Conclusions and Recommendations, 97

6   EPIDEMIOLOGY OF WOMEN'S DRINKING   100
    Methodologic Considerations, 101
    Definitions and Patterns of Drinking Among U.S. Women, 105
    Needed Research on Pregnant Women's Drinking, 107
    Conclusions and Recommendations, 109

7   PREVENTION OF FETAL ALCOHOL SYNDROME   112
    A Public Health Model of Prevention, 113
    Universal Prevention Interventions, 116
    Selective Prevention Interventions, 120
    Indicated Prevention Interventions, 135
    Maintenance and Aftercare, 142
    Program Evaluation, 142
    Public Health Service-Funded Research, 144
    Summary, 145
    Recommendations, 146

8   THE AFFECTED INDIVIDUAL: CLINICAL
    PRESENTATION, INTERVENTION, AND TREATMENT   154
    Clinical Issues in Individuals with FAS, ARBD, or ARND, 156
    Intervention and Prevention of Secondary Disabilities, 173
    Limitations and Barriers to the Provision of Services, 181

Summary: Intervention and Treatment, 184
Recommendations, 185

9   INTEGRATION AND COORDINATION: A CONCLUDING
    COMMENT AND RECOMMENDATION   194

APPENDIX: BIOGRAPHIES   197

INDEX   203

FETAL ALCOHOL SYNDROME

Executive Summary

Fetal alcohol syndrome (FAS), first described in the published medical literature in 1968, refers to a constellation of physical abnormalities, most obvious in the features of the face and in the reduced size of the newborn, and problems of behavior and cognition, in children born to mothers who drank heavily during pregnancy. These latter features lead to the most concern. The costs of FAS and related conditions can be quite high—for the individual, for the family, and for society. Rates of FAS in several of the most complete studies are similar—on the order of 0.5 to 3 cases per 1,000 births. Assuming an annual birth cohort of approximately 4 million, this translates into 2 to 12 thousand FAS births per year in this country. These incidence figures are offered not as established facts but to emphasize the magnitude of a problem that has serious implications—for the individual and for society.

In recognition of the seriousness of this problem, the U.S. Congress mandated in Section 705 of Public Law 102-321, the ADAMHA Reorganization Act, that the Institute of Medicine (IOM) of the National Academy of Sciences conduct a study of FAS and related birth defects. This report is in response to that mandate.

The charge to the committee was to improve the understanding of available research knowledge and experience on:

- tools and approaches for diagnosing FAS and related disorders,
- the prevalence of FAS and related disorders in the general population of the United States,
- the effectiveness of surveillance systems, and

1

• the availability and effectiveness of prevention and treatment programs for these conditions.

As part of its work, the committee reviewed and assessed U.S. Department of Health and Human Services agency research on the topic and provided guidance for the future.

FAS is caused by prenatal exposure to high levels of alcohol. FAS is not a "drunk" baby or a baby physically dependent on or addicted to alcohol. Although the manifestations of FAS might change with age, FAS never completely disappears and, as with many developmental disabilities, there is no cure, although there might be some amelioration in some individuals. The committee studied data on the relation between low or moderate levels of prenatal alcohol exposure and more subtle abnormalities associated with such exposure, but it was unable to conclude that these subtle abnormalities, as detected by statistical calculations from epidemiologic studies of defined populations, do or do not represent a distinct clinical entity. The clinical significance of these effects for an individual is not clear. The committee is cognizant of the grave concern of many pregnant or preconceptional women and their partners about possible effects of less than heavy consumption of alcohol. The lack of diagnostic criteria for or more definitive statements regarding possible effects of low to moderate exposure to alcohol should not be interpreted as contradictory to the Surgeon General's warning against drinking alcohol during pregnancy.

DIAGNOSIS AND CLINICAL EVALUATION OF FETAL ALCOHOL SYNDROME

A medical diagnosis serves several major purposes: to facilitate communication among clinicians; to facilitate communication between clinician and patient (including, in this instance, the parents of patients); to assist in the study of pathophysiology and etiology; and to guide treatment. In addition to the well-documented guidelines of good reliability and validity, a number of practical considerations also inform decisions about diagnostic criteria. Placing a patient in a diagnostic category confers both benefits and disabilities. For example, the diagnosis of FAS may validate a patient's disability and facilitate appropriate interventions and social benefits. On the other hand, the diagnosis may also be used to stigmatize and to create self-fulfilling prophecies about the future that could be detrimental to the patient and his or her family.

The key issues noted by the committee for identification of FAS include the following:

1. Should a documented history of exposure to alcohol be required for the diagnosis of FAS?
2. Which physical features should be used to define the disorder?

3. Can behavioral or cognitive features be used to define the disorder?

4. Is there a role for ancillary measures (e.g., magnetic resonance imaging [MRI]) in making the diagnosis?

5. Can criteria be designed to be used across the life span?

6. What is the relationship of so-called fetal alcohol effects to fetal alcohol syndrome?

The committee studied the previous diagnostic criteria and felt that some of the issues confusing the clinical and research communities could be resolved with fairly minor changes (Table 1). The committee delineates five diagnostic categories. The rubric of Fetal Alcohol Syndrome contains criteria for (Category 1) FAS with a history of maternal alcohol exposure, (Category 2) FAS without a history of maternal alcohol exposure, and (Category 3) partial FAS with a history of maternal alcohol exposure. The naming of this diagnostic category was challenging for the committee, who found no perfect solution. The committee intends for this diagnostic category to include people with signs and symptoms attributable to significant prenatal alcohol exposure and who need medical, social services, and other attention. "Partial" denotes, to some people, that the condition might not be as severe, which the committee did not wish to imply. The committee settled on the use of "partial" despite these reservations.

Category 3 allows an FAS diagnosis to be given to someone who would not receive a Category 1 diagnosis, FAS with confirmed maternal alcohol exposure. A Category 3 diagnosis could be particularly useful, for example, for some patients who present for diagnosis as an adult. The natural history of FAS is such that some of the "hallmark" indicators used in infancy or childhood are not maintained into adolescence or adulthood. This diagnosis can also be used as a "holding" category as a means to defer a diagnosis of Category 1, FAS with confirmed maternal history of alcohol exposure, until more data collection or evaluation, including documentation as to whether behavioral and cognitive abnormalities persist over time, can support a more definitive diagnosis. In the newborn, for example, there is some controversy whether some behavioral abnormalities, such as abnormalities of state regulation, indicate or predict long-term dysfunction due to fetal alcohol exposure. In such cases, documentation of abnormalities over time would be important.

The committee has defined two other diagnostic categories: Category 4, alcohol-related birth defects (ARBD; physical anomalies only), and Category 5, alcohol-related neurodevelopmental disorder (ARND). Diagnostic categories 4 and 5 include clinical conditions for which clinical or animal research has linked maternal alcohol ingestion to an observed outcome. These final two diagnostic categories are intended to represent some degree of uncertainty whether prenatal alcohol exposure caused the adverse effects documented in an individual patient, or whether other factors were causative in this case. Because of the variability in the specific presentation of FAS, ARBD, or ARND, these diagnoses are most

TABLE 1   Diagnostic Criteria for Fetal Alcohol Syndrome (FAS) and
Alcohol-Related Effects

Fetal Alcohol Syndrome

1. FAS with confirmed maternal alcohol exposure[a]

A. Confirmed maternal alcohol exposure[a]

B. Evidence of a characteristic pattern of facial anomalies that includes features such as
short palpebral fissures and abnormalities in the premaxillary zone (e.g., flat upper lip,
flattened philtrum, and flat midface)

C. Evidence of growth retardation, as in at least one of the following:
  — low birth weight for gestational age
  — decelerating weight over time not due to nutrition
  — disproportional low weight to height

D. Evidence of CNS neurodevelopmental abnormalities, as in at least one of the following:
  — decreased cranial size at birth
  — structural brain abnormalities (e.g., microcephaly, partial or complete agenesis of the
corpus callosum, cerebellar hypoplasia)
  — neurological hard or soft signs (as age appropriate), such as impaired fine motor skills,
neurosensory hearing loss, poor tandem gait, poor eye-hand coordination

2. FAS without confirmed maternal alcohol exposure

B, C, and D as above

3. Partial FAS with confirmed maternal alcohol exposure

A. Confirmed maternal alcohol exposure[a]

B. Evidence of some components of the pattern of characteristic facial anomalies

Either C or D or E

C. Evidence of growth retardation, as in at least one of the following:
  — low birth weight for gestational age
  — decelerating weight over time not due to nutrition
  — disproportional low weight to height

D. Evidence of CNS neurodevelopmental abnormalities, as in:
  — decreased cranial size at birth
  — structural brain abnormalities (e.g., microcephaly, partial or complete agenesis of the
corpus callosum, cerebellar hypoplasia)
  — neurological hard or soft signs (as age appropriate) such as impaired fine motor skills,
neurosensory hearing loss, poor tandem gait, poor eye-hand coordination

E. Evidence of a complex pattern of behavior or cognitive abnormalities that are inconsistent
with developmental level and cannot be explained by familial background or environment
alone, such as learning difficulties; deficits in school performance; poor impulse control;
problems in social perception; deficits in higher level receptive and expressive language;
poor capacity for abstraction or metacognition; specific deficits in mathematical skills; or
problems in memory, attention, or judgment

Alcohol-Related Effects

Clinical conditions in which there is a history of maternal alcohol exposure,[a,b] and where
clinical or animal research has linked maternal alcohol ingestion to an observed outcome.
There are two categories, which may co-occur. If both diagnoses are present, then both
diagnoses should be rendered:

TABLE 1 Continued

Alcohol-Related Effects (continued)

4. Alcohol-related birth defects (ARBD)

List of congenital anomalies, including malformations and dysplasias

Cardiac	Atrial septal defects	Aberrant great vessels
	Ventricular septal defects	Tetralogy of Fallot
Skeletal	Hypoplastic nails	Clinodactyly
	Shortened fifth digits	Pectus excavatum and carinatum
	Radioulnar synostosis	Klippel-Feil syndrome
	Flexion contractures	Hemivertebrae
	Camptodactyly	Scoliosis
Renal	Aplastic, dysplastic,	Ureteral duplications
	hypoplastic kidneys	Hydronephrosis
	Horseshoe kidneys	
Ocular	Strabismus	Refractive problems secondary to small globes
	Retinal vascular anomalies	
Auditory	Conductive hearing loss	Neurosensory hearing loss
Other	Virtually every malformation has been described in some patient with FAS. The etiologic specificity of most of these anomalies to alcohol teratogenesis remains uncertain.	

5. Alcohol-related neurodevelopmental disorder (ARND)

Presence of:

A. Evidence of CNS neurodevelopmental abnormalities, as in any one of the following:

— decreased cranial size at birth

— structural brain abnormalities (e.g., microcephaly, partial or complete agenesis of the corpus callosum, cerebellar hypoplasia)

— neurological hard or soft signs (as age appropriate), such as impaired fine motor skills, neurosensory hearing loss, poor tandem gait, poor eye-hand coordination

and/or:

B. Evidence of a complex pattern of behavior or cognitive abnormalities that are inconsistent with developmental level and cannot be explained by familial background or environment alone, such as learning difficulties; deficits in school performance; poor impulse control; problems in social perception; deficits in higher level receptive and expressive language; poor capacity for abstraction or metacognition; specific deficits in mathematical skills; or problems in memory, attention, or judgment

---

aA pattern of excessive intake characterized by substantial, regular intake or heavy episodic drinking. Evidence of this pattern may include frequent episodes of intoxication, development of tolerance or withdrawal, social problems related to drinking, legal problems related to drinking, engaging in physically hazardous behavior while drinking, or alcohol-related medical problems such as hepatic disease.

bAs further research is completed and as, or if, lower quantities or variable patterns of alcohol use are associated with ARBD or ARND, these patterns of alcohol use should be incorporated into the diagnostic criteria.

valuable clinically if accompanied by a description of the specific problems experienced at the time by the patient.

All diagnoses but Category 2, FAS without confirmed history of maternal alcohol exposure, require a history of maternal alcohol exposure. The committee defined the relevant history of maternal exposure as a pattern of excessive intake characterized by substantial, regular intake or heavy episodic drinking. As further research is completed and as, or if, lower quantities or variable patterns of alcohol use are associated with ARBD or ARND, these patterns of alcohol use should be incorporated into the diagnostic criteria.

Key Recommendations

Research recommendations include

- research to evaluate the utility, reliability, and validity of this scheme for classification and diagnosis;
- research, both cross-sectional and longitudinal, to assess the characteristics and clinical expression of these syndromes across the life span, particularly after adolescence;
- investigation of the differences in expression and specificity of behavioral and cognitive deficits in FAS and ARND;
- further clinical research, as well as research using animal models, to examine the adverse developmental effects of prenatal alcohol exposure, and to develop more specific biologic markers for diagnosis (e.g., biomarkers to confirm maternal alcohol exposure, endocrine signals, imaging techniques).

EPIDEMIOLOGY AND SURVEILLANCE OF FAS, ARBD, AND ARND

The success of any public health program can be measured by comparing the incidence or prevalence of a particular societal problem before that program was implemented with its incidence or prevalence after implementation. Such data are also important for estimating the societal impact of these disorders and are crucial at the initial stages of planning, organizing, and implementing prevention programs aimed at the general population as well as at specific at-risk populations.

The literature on the prevalence and epidemiology of FAS is far from consistent or conclusive. A limited proportion of mothers who are very heavy drinkers will have children with FAS. Various studies reporting the occurrence of FAS range from 0.5 to 3 births per 1,000 in most populations, with some communities having much higher rates. FAS and other diagnosable ARBDs or ARNDs may occur more frequently.

Passive surveillance is the strategy generally used to monitor birth defects.

A national passive surveillance system that includes FAS uses hospital discharge data on both live and stillborn newborns and has estimated the incidence of FAS at 3.7 per 10,000 births for 1992. Although passive surveillance is relatively inexpensive, it is notoriously inaccurate; given that FAS is a complex diagnosis, it may go unrecognized at birth. Thus, registry-based estimates of FAS prevalence can be expected to be gross underestimates. Data obtained passively from clinic-based studies, whether based on prospective epidemiologic studies or retrospectively of children referred for clinical evaluation, typically result in numbers that are higher than prevalence estimates derived by using standard surveillance methodologies.

Active surveillance involves direct prospective collection of data using experimentally driven protocols rather than using available data such as medical charts. Two classic types of active surveillance are prospective epidemiologic studies of the infant outcomes associated with maternal alcohol use and population-based active FAS case ascertainment. In general, these rates are higher by an order of magnitude than those estimated from passive surveillance studies. These studies can be very expensive and labor intensive. The populations studied in epidemiologic studies of maternal alcohol abuse frequently do not include sufficient women who abuse alcohol at levels that produce offspring with FAS. Population-based studies can assist in addressing some of the criticisms of passive surveillance systems and may be useful for linking identified individuals to treatment programs and for evaluating comprehensive prevention efforts.

An alternative to passively monitoring the incidence of FAS at birth is to develop proxy measures of FAS, such as one facial anomaly and one indicator of growth deficiency, and use these as surveillance criteria for active case ascertainment that would identify a group of newborns with a high probability of having FAS. One would then need to develop a means to estimate from these kinds of data an approximation of the incidence or prevalence of FAS. Population-based studies in a variety of populations might be useful in determining such an estimation factor.

Key Conclusions and Recommendations

The committee concludes that FAS, ARBD, and ARND are a completely preventable set of birth defects and neurodevelopmental abnormalities, that FAS is arguably the most common known nongenetic cause of mental retardation, and that FAS, ARBD, and ARND constitute a major public health concern. To address the lack of baseline data and the wide variation of prevalence estimates for subpopulations, including ethnic minorities, the committee recommends that:

• an interagency plan be developed for a national survey to estimate the prevalence and incidence of FAS, ARND, and ARBD, which could utilize active surveillance techniques;

• improved data collection and surveillance be implemented to identify specifically children with FAS, ARND, and ARBD in various social and educational environments (e.g., maternal and child health block grant programs, Head Start programs, and Early Intervention and Special Education Services); and

• when active surveillance strategies are employed that identify children with FAS, ARND, or ARBD, appropriate linkages should be in place among agencies and local clinics to facilitate treatment.

EPIDEMIOLOGY AND SURVEILLANCE OF DRINKING DURING PREGNANCY

Approximately 60 percent of adult women in the United States drink alcohol at least occasionally. Approximately 4 percent of women would be considered to have alcohol abuse or alcohol dependence, as defined by the fourth edition of the Diagnostic and Statistical Manual (DSM-IV). Available data indicate substantially lower rates of both drinking (approximately 20 percent according to national surveys) and heavy drinking (less than 1 percent) among pregnant women, relative to nonpregnant women of childbearing age. (By comparison, a national survey estimates that 20 percent of pregnant women smoked, 5.5 percent used any illicit drugs, 0.9 percent used crack cocaine, and 10 percent used psychotherapeutics for medically-indicated conditions.) Although the percentages are small in *relative* terms, the large *absolute numbers* of women who continue to engage in heavy and hazardous drinking throughout pregnancy make it imperative to understand the personal and social factors that make women more likely to continue drinking heavily during pregnancy.

Although researchers have seen some encouraging changes in drinking patterns during pregnancy over the years, there is no substantive evidence of any change in drinking behavior among women who drink more heavily or abuse alcohol, either in terms of proportions of heavy drinkers at the time of conception or in terms of consumption levels during pregnancy.

Current clinic-based studies of drinking in pregnant women include relatively small numbers of women who are heavier drinkers, alcohol abusers, or alcohol dependent and few studies of drinking during pregnancy assess personality or social-environmental variables associated with drinking. Because only a small percentage of women are pregnant at any point, only general population surveys with very large samples will allow reliable analysis of drinking correlates among women pregnant at the time of the survey.

Key Recommendations

Therefore, the committee recommends special attention to the following research questions and issues:

• expansion of studies of pregnant women, where possible, to include measurement of psychological, social-environmental, dietary, and other factors that may influence women's drinking behavior or fetal outcome;
• inclusion of questions regarding alcohol consumption and pregnancy status in appropriate future national health surveys;
• focus on protective factors that may decrease women's drinking or prevent fetal injury from alcohol consumption;
• continued and increased epidemiological study of women's drinking patterns, including efforts to maximize the validity of self-report measures, efforts which could include the use, where and when appropriate, of a biomarker for alcohol exposure.

PREVENTION

Because prenatal alcohol exposure most likely is associated with a spectrum of effects ranging from negligible to severe, a number of different drinking patterns with various characteristics and etiologies need to be addressed. Cultural, sociological, behavioral, public health, and medical disciplines are relevant to the prevention of FAS and related conditions.

The committee thought about the prevention of FAS and related problems within a conceptual framework that would encompass a broad spectrum of prevention measures and that acknowledges that prevention of FAS includes treatment and maintenance for alcohol abuse in the mother. A woman's partner and her community are appropriate targets for preventive interventions and subjects for preventive intervention research. After the birth of an FAS child, there are two targets for intervention—the mother and the child. Each of them is a patient in need of care; each is a target for treatment and maintenance to improve their health and well-being as well as for preventive intervention for the birth of another FAS child. The hallmark of this framework is that one enters into the continuum of interventions in a manner proportional to the certainty and severity of the risk involved. That is, the intervention becomes more specific and intensive as the risk is defined less by general population characteristics and more by individual characteristics.

Universal prevention intervention strives to ensure that all members of society understand that drinking alcohol can have hazardous consequences, particularly during pregnancy. The universal prevention message for FAS is a conservative one that encourages abstinence prior to conception and throughout pregnancy as the safest alternative. One of the basic techniques used in universal prevention is public education. Visits to family practitioners and to obstetrician gynecologists offer the opportunity for brief messages about the importance of responsible alcohol use and for providing general information about the risks of alcohol to the fetus.

Selective prevention interventions target people who are at greater risk for a particular outcome because they are members of a subgroup known to be at higher risk than the general population. These interventions involve different levels of targeting and intensity compared to universal preventive interventions. Targets of selective prevention for FAS, ARBD, and ARND include women who drink alcohol and are in the reproductive age range and their partners. Although paternal alcohol exposure does not cause FAS, the important supportive role that the male partner plays in a healthy pregnancy is well established and cannot be emphasized too strongly. However, many women who are at high risk for FAS are unmarried, in very unstable relationships, or both.

Physicians or other health care providers should be prepared to talk to women about their alcohol use, screen women for indication of alcohol abuse, conduct further assessments as necessary, and be prepared to offer brief interventions. If appropriate, referral for formal treatment of alcohol dependence should be made. In general, the strength of the intervention should be proportional to the level of risk. There are studies showing that some pregnant women who drink moderately or heavily are amenable to interventions offered in conjunction with prenatal care. However, there are no consistent data to predict who will respond to such interventions and who will continue to drink.

Indicated prevention interventions target high-risk individuals. A small proportion of women within some populations give birth to most of the FAS children. The committee therefore considers the target for indicated prevention interventions to be a woman who engages in heavy drinking while pregnant or at risk for being pregnant, particularly a pregnant or preconceptional woman who drinks alcohol and who has already given birth to a child with FAS, ARBD, or ARND. As with selective interventions, the committee would also include interventions aimed at the partner, significant friends, or family members of a woman who fits the profile just described. Indicated *prevention* of FAS includes *treatment* for alcohol abuse or dependence for a pregnant woman or for a woman highly likely to become pregnant. The committee identified little controlled research into the most effective ways to treat pregnant women who drink.

Because, in many cases, women do not seek obstetric services until delivery, any health care provider who comes in contact with women who abuse alcohol should consider brief intervention therapies and referral to more formal alcohol abuse treatment, if appropriate. Women of reproductive age who abuse alcohol should also be offered referral and access to birth control information and services.

For the comparatively small group of women who continue to drink heavily during pregnancy, formal treatment of alcohol dependence may be needed. Treatment programs described are typically broad, multimodal interventions that are intended to address the complex problems exhibited by this population. However, systematic data collection on characteristics of women who drink heavily during pregnancy has been rare. Thus, treatment programs for pregnant women who abuse alcohol have been based primarily on the availability of services and on clinical judgment, and in the relative absence of empirical data that could inform the conceptualization and development of treatments targeted to address the specific problems of this population.

The literature in recent years suggest that one effective way to help alcohol-abusing women who had FAS children might be through intensive case management. Case management involves all members of the extended family and should include enlisting the positive action of the male partner. Children benefit from such efforts, too. Often children of FAS-producing mothers are in foster placement because of neglect or abuse. A major motivator for maintenance and aftercare is to improve the social and health status of the mother so that she can regain or retain custody of her children.

Key Recommendations

- The committee recommends that until such time as clear dose-response relationships are established, pregnant women and those about to become pregnant be counseled to avoid alcohol consumption throughout pregnancy.
- The committee recommends greatly increased attention among sponsors of prevention initiatives, independent of the target population, to evaluating the effectiveness of programs implemented. This recommendation applies to all levels of prevention interventions.
- The committee recommends that research efforts include comparisons of prevention methods at all levels in order to provide information to policy makers about relative costs and benefits.

Indicated Prevention Interventions

- The committee recommends that a high priority be placed on research efforts to design, implement, and evaluate prevention interventions that can effectively guide pregnant women who drink heavily to alcohol treatment. Research or programs should also include:

- assessment of methods to involve women's partners and family members in interventions to decrease or stop drinking;
- implementation of appropriate screening tools, including biomarkers of alcohol exposure, to identify women who are drinking moderate to heavy amounts of alcohol during pregnancy;
- incorporation of comprehensive reproductive counseling and contraceptive services in prevention and treatment programs for substance-abusing women;
- development of training programs for professionals in the identification of heavy drinking, and referral to appropriate regional centers or prevention services;
- basic research in animal models to elucidate further the mechanisms of

alcohol teratogenesis, which might lead to pharmacologic or other strategies for amelioration of the effects of alcohol exposure in utero.

Selective Prevention Interventions

• The committee recommends increased research efforts to design, implement, and evaluate selective prevention interventions to decrease risks of FAS, ARND, and ARBD through programs aimed toward women who are pregnant or may become pregnant, and who drink alcohol.

• Where the utility of specific intervention programs has been established, the committee recommends broad implementation of successful prevention interventions. Programs developed or studied should include the following:

— intervention targeted to specific demographic groups that have been demonstrated to be at higher risk for FAS, ARBD, and ARND, as well as those who exhibit risk factors associated with moderate to heavy alcohol consumption during pregnancy.

Universal Prevention Interventions

• The committee recommends that although data are insufficient regarding the effectiveness of universal prevention interventions, such interventions should be continued to raise awareness about the risks of FAS, ARBD, and ARND. However, the most important approach to universal prevention is probably the development of a medical environment in which concepts of the risk of FAS, ARBD, and ARND are incorporated into routine health care.

TREATMENT OF THE AFFECTED INDIVIDUAL

Many prenatally-exposed individuals do not receive correct diagnosis or treatment for their alcohol-related disabilities. There has been a curious lack of enthusiasm for targeted efforts directed at the prevention of secondary disabilities. The view that intervention may not be useful in children affected by alcohol is inconsistent with the attitude taken toward other groups of high-risk and disabled children. Few systematic attempts have been made to intervene with alcohol-affected children to test the possibility that such strategies would be effective in producing more positive outcomes.

In understanding how to meet the needs of individuals with FAS, it is first necessary to describe the behavioral characteristics of affected children as well as the social environment in which many affected children live. Information about affected children is derived mainly from two sources: (1) retrospective and uncontrolled, descriptive clinical studies of clinically referred children with FAS and fetal alcohol effects, and (2) prospective research studies of children exposed to alcohol in utero due to maternal drinking. In most such prospective studies, maternal drinking is in the light to moderate range, with only a few women drinking in the heavy range. As a result, most of the children in these prospective studies are not dysmorphic and would not, therefore, qualify for a diagnosis of FAS, although in some cases they may have milder effects that are observable through focused testing or the statistical analysis of group data.

For the clinician, as well as the research scientist, there are several important questions that must be answered in order to plan interventions for individuals with FAS, partial FAS and possible ARND. The first question is whether there are discernible patterns in the development of prenatally exposed children. A review of existing information about the development of these children suggests the following conclusions: *The data base is limited. There is a great deal of variability in outcome. Early identification is possible in some cases. Effects of prenatal exposure appear to become more significant later in the child's development, perhaps due to the nature of a disorder that may affect behaviors associated with more mature social functioning.*

The second significant question is whether developmental problems seen in alcohol-exposed children should be attributed solely to the effects of the teratogen on neurological functioning, solely to the effects of environmental factors such as social class and dysfunctional families, or to some combination of the two. At present, there is no easy answer to this question. Because children develop within a family and a community, their caregiving environment must be given careful consideration as well. However, the social and environmental factors that may affect the development of individuals with FAS or ARND have not been adequately investigated.

Anecdotal evidence suggests that children with FAS, ARBD, or ARND are more likely to have negative caregiving environments than are typical children or children with other disabilities. The first risk for these children is loss of their biological parents. Clinical observation also suggests that children with FAS or possible alcohol-related effects often come to the attention of protective service agencies and frequently may enter foster care or be placed for adoption. Some children receive a stable placement; others are shifted repeatedly because their behavior is hard for some foster or adoptive families to manage.

The third question concerns specificity. It is not clear that the behaviors reportedly shown by alcohol-affected individuals are different from those shown by other persons who are mentally retarded, have specific learning disabilities, are diagnosed with ADHD, or have been reared in dysfunctional families. Rarely have these groups been compared to other clinically diagnosed groups to identify factors specific to those who have been exposed to alcohol. If it is true that there are specific problems in children with FAS and ARND, it may be possible to design targeted prevention efforts that will help to avoid the more negative outcomes that have been observed.

Although in some cases the prenatal exposure may have had permanent effects, it still might be possible to avoid the development of secondary disabilities in these individuals by early identification and appropriate treatment over the life span. There is no systematically compiled information available describing the number of people with FAS receiving services or the kinds of services received by individuals with FAS or other alcohol-related deficits. At the present time, there are no empirical studies available of the effects of educational intervention, either generalized (the standard services offered to all qualifying children) or specific (programs specifically designed for those with FAS or ARBD), on alcohol-affected children. Faced with a lack of published information about teaching methods and the effectiveness of treatment for alcohol-exposed children, some teachers and parents have turned to the "wisdom of practice." When these teachers' methods are examined, it is clear that their suggestions are well grounded in an understanding of young children and in practical knowledge about teaching. It is not clear, however, that these methods are of relatively greater value in alcohol-affected children than in other groups. However, to determine whether they are more or less effective with children with fetal alcohol effects, evaluation of methods and programs will be required.

In addition to medical and educational interventions directed at affected individuals, other strategies have been considered to improve outcomes for alcohol-affected children and adults. Research suggests that few professionals working with children have adequate training in identifying and treating the effects of fetal alcohol exposure in children, although some programs that have provided professional education have been successful. Because the child is being reared within a family, whether the biological family or an adoptive or foster family, intervention for the prevention of secondary disabilities in alcohol-affected children must address the needs of the family as well. The way in which this support is provided will depend on the age of the child and the kind of family situation that exists.

Key Recommendations

The committee concludes that there are no specific programs to treat children with FAS, ARBD, or ARND, and other efforts to prevent secondary disability in these children are insufficient and inadequate. Given the known value of early intervention for other conditions, however, it is important to identify children with FAS, ARBD, or ARND as early as possible. Thus, in the committee's view, action to bring needed programs and efforts to an acceptable level must proceed on a number of fronts. The committee, therefore, recommends the following actions to address these needs:

• Clusters of high-quality diagnostic and treatment services should be available locally and regionally.
• Programs serving children with FAS, ARND, or ARBD should meet the

special, complex needs of such children, including consideration of the families involved and increased availability of parenting training for caretakers (birth parents, foster parents, and adoptive parents).

• Educational materials should be developed for professionals who deal with school-age children to increase their awareness of FAS, ARND, or ARBD as a potential cause of ADHD-like behaviors, including hyperactivity, and to facilitate their referral of such children to other appropriate or needed services.

• Clinical practice guidelines should be developed for follow-up and treatment of children with FAS, ARND, or ARBD.

A necessary complement to the above actions is an expanded knowledge base. The committee, thus, views further research as essential to providing adequate treatment of children affected by FAS, ARND, and ARBD. The committee recommends additional research in the following areas:

• research to distinguish the role of the postnatal environment in modifying the effects of fetal alcohol exposure, including research on adopted versus non-adopted children with these disorders;

• research on the social and emotional status of school age children affected by FAS, ARND, or ARBD and research on the existence of specific impairments associated with these syndromes, particularly impairments in attention, language, sensory integration, and other behavioral problems;

• evaluation of the effectiveness of educational interventions on children with FAS, ARND, or ARBD, possibly beginning with the examination of educational interventions that look promising in case studies or in studies of children exposed to illicit drugs in utero.

INTEGRATION AND COORDINATION

There is no single, organized discipline within medicine that can, at this time, logically be held responsible or accountable for the development of a comprehensive approach to preventing and treating fetal alcohol syndrome (FAS), alcohol-related birth defects (ARBD), or alcohol-related neurodevelopmental disorder (ARND). Nor is there a single discipline in the broader arena of health and health care appropriate for this role. No group has yet shown any interest in the management of FAS, ARBD, or ARND patients as adults. Therefore, these disorders lie within the purview of many groups but are clearly not the full responsibility of any one. Like any problem that falls between organized disciplines, progress is unavoidably hampered. Both FAS research and service delivery suffer.

Such structural marginalization is also evident in government, where it is difficult to find a local, state, or federal government system that is positioned to address these disorders in a comprehensive manner. It is clear that neither governmental structures nor the organization of modern medicine and health care can be redesigned. Thus, the challenge is to improve communication and cooperation among health, education, developmental disabilities, and social services disciplines and government agencies.

RECOMMENDATION

Therefore, the committee recommends that an interagency task force, or other entity comprised of representatives from the relevant federal research, surveillance, and services agencies, be established to coordinate national efforts in FAS, ARBD, and ARND. Lead responsibility for heading this task force should be assigned to NIAAA, because it is experienced at encouraging research and at incorporating research methodologies into all activities and has had the longest history in addressing FAS. However, all member agencies should be willing and able to translate research findings into service delivery and policy development activities and be expected to contribute to and be consulted with about achieving the overall goals of preventing and treating FAS.

It is suggested that one of the top priorities of such a coordinating body should be to forge interagency cooperation in the adoption of a common terminology and set of definitions related to these disorders, such as proposed in this report, and the design and implementation of national surveys to estimate the true prevalence of FAS, ARND, and ARBD. At the same time, prevention and treatment of secondary disabilities associated with FAS, ARND, and ARBD, as well as prevention and treatment of alcohol abuse and dependence by pregnant women and by women at risk of becoming pregnant, should be a high, and long-term, priority of this coordinating body. Additional important areas of focus should include consideration of basic research and communication among the basic and clinical research communities and the health services community. Recommendations for research in all aspects of FAS can be found in this report and should serve as guidance for the coordinating body. Finally, the coordinating body should take active steps to encourage and facilitate the rigorous evaluation of all intervention programs.

1

Introduction

It sounds simple: women who drink excessively while pregnant are at high risk for giving birth to children with birth defects. Therefore, to prevent these defects, women should stop drinking alcohol during all phases of pregnancy. Alternatively, women who drink alcohol should not become pregnant unless and until they can control their drinking. More than 20 years ago, when fetal alcohol syndrome (FAS) was first described in the published medical literature, there were high hopes for its prevention. In fact, this has not been simple, and the biomedical and public health communities are still struggling to eliminate a birth defect that should be absolutely preventable.

HISTORY

Although references to the effects of prenatal exposure to alcohol can be found in classical and biblical literature, fetal alcohol syndrome was first described in the medical literature in France by Lemoine et al. in 1968. Researchers in the United States soon also published a landmark report describing a constellation of birth defects in children born to alcoholic women (Jones and Smith, 1973). FAS has since been described in most countries of the world. Briefly, FAS refers to a constellation of physical abnormalities, most obvious in the features of the face (see Figure 1-1) and in the reduced size of the newborn, and problems of behavior and cognition. These latter features lead to the most concern.

The degree of abnormality in any one measure can vary greatly between individuals and can change with time in the same individual. For example,

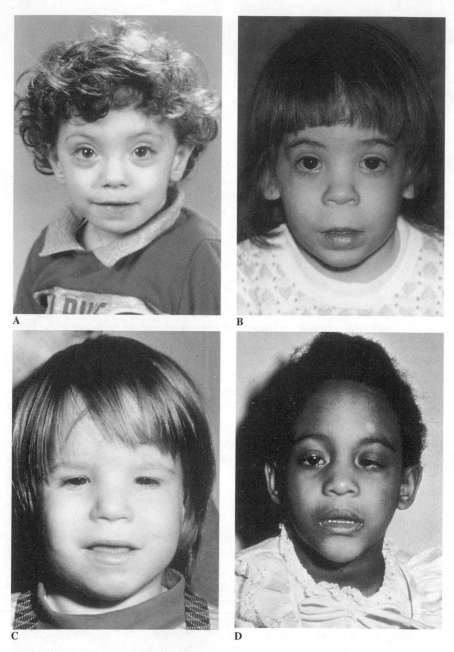

A

B

C

D

FIGURE 1-1 Photographs of children with fetal alcohol syndrome. SOURCES: Figures 4C and 4D: Reprinted with permission from Jones et al. (1973). Copyright 1973 by the Lancet Ltd. Figure 4B: Reprinted with permission from Clarren and Smith (1978). Copyright 1978 by the New England Journal of Medicine, Massachusetts Medical Society.

people diagnosed with FAS can have IQs from well within the normal range to the severely mentally retarded range. The physical anomalies can be slight or quite striking. Some people with FAS live fairly normal lives if given adequate and structured support throughout their lives, whereas others are severely impaired. The defects may or may not be apparent or easily diagnosed at birth. Although the manifestations of the damage might change with age, FAS never completely disappears and, as with many developmental disabilities, there is no cure, although there might be some amelioration in some individuals. FAS does not refer to signs of acute alcohol exposure or withdrawal at birth. Newborns can have blood alcohol levels high enough to affect acutely their central nervous system function and not have FAS. Newborns can also have no alcohol in their bloodstream *at time of delivery* but still have FAS. FAS is not a "drunk" baby.

The costs of FAS and related conditions can be quite high—for the individual, for the family, and for society. Three groups have tried to estimate these costs, and these estimates vary greatly (Bloss, 1994). These estimates are problematic, because of uncertainties regarding the incidence and prevalence of FAS and uncertainties related to the full extent of health (and other) problems experienced throughout the lifetime of people with FAS. Estimates of the occurrence of FAS in North American communities range from 0 per 1,000 (incidence; Abel and Sokol, 1987, 1991) to 120 per 1,000 (prevalence; Robinson et al., 1987), although rates in several of the most complete studies are similar—on the order of 0.5 to 3 cases per 1,000 births. Assuming an annual birth cohort of approximately 4 million, this translates into 2 to 12 thousand FAS births per year in this country. As described in the report, there is a lack of longitudinal data on the extent of possible problems of adults with FAS. Therefore, cost estimates for the United States range from $75 million (Abel and Sokol, 1991) to $9.7 billion (Harwood and Napolitano, 1985). The total lifetime cost per typical case of FAS for a child born in 1980 was estimated to be $596,000 undiscounted[1] (Harwood and Napolitano, 1985). These incidence and cost figures are offered not as established facts but they are intended to emphasize that regardless of the details, or any one specific estimate, the costs of FAS to the individual and society are high.

Since publication of the papers by Lemoine and by Jones and Smith, the biomedical, public health, research, and public policy communities have devoted much time and energy to a fascinating problem of teratology (the study of the effects of chemical exposure on the developing fetus), neurobiology, disease prevention, and social disarray. The U.S. Public Health Service has spent millions of dollars in research, public education, and service programs related to the

---

[1]Discounting is a tool used in economic analyses to assign smaller weights to costs incurred in the distant future. Undiscounted amounts represent simple sums, regardless of when the costs would be incurred.

topic. Important concepts have been established through research. For example, well-controlled research studies on rats, mice, and nonhuman primates has demonstrated that alcohol exposure causes FAS. However, while alcohol is the necessary teratogen, it alone may not be sufficient to produce FAS in humans or birth defects in animals. As with most teratogens, not every fetus exposed to significant amounts of alcohol is affected. The outcomes might be modulated by numerous biologic and environmental factors, such as nutrition, threshold, timing, genetic susceptibility, pattern of alcohol exposure, or fetal resilience. Further research is needed to fully elucidate the factors that influence the expression of alcohol teratogenesis.

Public education campaigns have taught many women and their partners, as well as the medical community and society at large, that excessive alcohol consumption is dangerous during pregnancy. Reduction in the occurrence of substance abuse during pregnancy, reduction in the incidence of FAS, and an increase in the questioning of patients by health care providers about alcohol and other drug use are goals of the Public Health Service's Healthy People 2000 initiative (U.S. Department of Health and Human Services, 1991). See Table 1-1.

Prevention of birth defects as a salient public health goal presents some exemplary success stories. A good example is the advocacy for and impact of rubella immunizations for children and women of childbearing age with no history of natural rubella or rubella immunization. An outbreak in the United States in the mid-1960s resulted in an estimated 20,000 children born with congenital rubella syndrome (CRS). CRS occurs in 20 to 25 percent of babies born to mothers who get rubella in the first trimester of pregnancy and results in congenital heart disease, deafness, mental retardation, and other fetal abnormalities. An estimate of the lifetime cost of CRS is about $330,000 per case. With widespread introduction of rubella vaccines in the late 1960s and the requirement for rubella immunization prior to school entry, the number of reported cases of CRS in the

TABLE 1-1 Examples of Healthy People 2000 Goals Relevant to Fetal Alcohol Syndrome (FAS)

Objective	1987 Baseline	Target 2000
Incidence of FAS (per 1,000 live births)	0.22	0.12
Abstinence from alcohol during pregnancy	79%	Increase by 20%
Screening by obstetrician/gynecologist for alcohol use	34%	75%
Referrals by obstetrician/gynecologist for alcohol treatment	24%	75%
Screening by obstetrician/gynecologist for drug use	32%	75%
Referrals by obstetrician/gynecologist for drug treatment	28%	75%

United States hit a low of 225 in 1988. As another example, new findings that folic acid deficiency during pregnancy can result in neural tube defects have led to recommendations that grain be fortified with folic acid to prevent these birth defects. Availability of effective prevention strategies led to public policy debates and recommendations for action.

The emergence of crack cocaine as a major medical and public health problem in the 1980s led to worries about a generation of crack babies who would cost the medical care system, primarily neonatal intensive care wards, huge amounts of money and who would overburden the education and social service systems with problems attributable to prenatal exposure to cocaine. Further research has shown that crack cocaine can lead to serious obstetrical complications and that some of the exposed newborns do have problems. Cocaine-exposed children have not been followed as extensively or for as long a time as alcohol-exposed children; what data have been published show some effects of prenatal cocaine exposure at three years of age, but the problems do not seem to be nearly as devastating as predicted, nor as severe as the long-term problems associated with alcohol exposure. In fact, some of the long-term effects associated with prenatal cocaine exposure may be due in part to the concurrent use of alcohol during pregnancy. The federal government invested millions of dollars in demonstration projects for services for substance-abusing women. Some of these programs included services for women who abuse alcohol, but the emphasis was usually on drugs, particularly illegal ones, other than alcohol, or on polydrug use. The attention to crack cocaine and its effects on the fetus is curious given that the percentage of pregnant women who drink (approximately 20 percent) far exceeds the percentage who use cocaine (approximately 1 percent; National Institute on Drug Abuse, 1994).

At the time, however, the cocaine epidemic and its potential risks to unborn children led to heated public policy debates. Policies of mandatory urine testing in delivery wards, and subsequent removal of a child from the care of a mother who tested positive for illegal substances, were instituted in many places (Blume, in press; Chavkin, 1990). The unintended negative consequences of these actions have led to a reconsideration and reversal of these policies more recently.

THE FEDERAL RESPONSIBILITY FOR FAS RESEARCH

As will be described in many parts of this report, FAS is a complicated health and social problem, involving many different sectors of the government. The U.S. Public Health Service (USPHS) contains the agencies with primary responsibility for research in the area. The National Institute on Alcohol Abuse and Alcoholism (NIAAA) of the National Institutes of Health (NIH) has the lead role in research on FAS. However, NIAAA is a relatively small institute of NIH. The NIAAA appropriation in 1993 was $177 million, compared with more than $400 million for the National Institute on Drug Abuse (NIDA) and slightly less than

$2 billion for the National Cancer Institute (U.S. Department of Health and Human Services, 1993). NIAAA programs related to FAS include very basic animal research, which has been the mainstay of research in this area; clinical and epidemiologic research on the effects of low to moderate alcohol use by pregnant women; and prevention research. The alcohol and pregnancy program at NIAAA included $9.8 million to $13.5 million for approximately 70 grants in each of fiscal years 1990-1994. Most of these research grants were RO1, investigator-initiated awards. NIAAA funds one fetal alcohol research center.

In addition, many research programs sponsored by NIAAA have ancillary importance to FAS, for example, the research it funds on the epidemiology of drinking by women or on general approaches to the prevention and treatment of alcohol abuse. As an example of the level of commitment by NIAAA to this issue, the prevention research program at NIAAA has ranged from $15 million to $19.8 million annually in recent years. As the lead research agency on alcohol, the institute and the USPHS can serve as a bully pulpit for the prevention of FAS and other alcohol-related problems. In fact, this has been the case. The U.S. Surgeon General first issued a warning against the dangers of alcohol during pregnancy in 1981. In addition to funding and conducting research, NIAAA publishes information for the public on FAS, sponsors research workshops on FAS, and has its staff speak at public meetings.

Other NIH institutes fund research relevant to, but not directly about, FAS. For example, NIDA funded a $4 million National Pregnancy and Health Survey on substance abuse, including alcohol, during pregnancy. The data on alcohol were a small part of the entire project. In addition, NIDA funds epidemiologic and clinical research on the effects of substance abuse during pregnancy, and alcohol is frequently one of the substances used by these populations. A rather large study funded by NIDA was the Perinatal 20 demonstration project assessing prevention of substance abuse during pregnancy. Although the major purpose was to look at the abuse of illegal substances, some data were collected on alcohol use, as well.

Another key USPHS agency involved in FAS work is the Centers for Disease Control and Prevention (CDC). The FAS Prevention Section is housed in CDC's National Center for Environmental Health, Division of Birth Defects and Developmental Disabilities. CDC's role is to collect data to define the scope of the problem; support the development and evaluation of FAS prevention projects; and build state capacity for coordinated, state-based FAS surveillance and prevention programs (CDC submission to IOM committee). The CDC maintains and analyzes surveillance programs that include FAS, such as the Birth Defects Monitoring Program. In addition, CDC sponsors and supports efforts to prevent FAS. The CDC currently has FAS prevention and surveillance projects supported through states and universities. As with NIAAA, CDC has ancillary programs related to maternal and child health, alcohol abuse, and epidemiologic surveillance that can support and inform FAS programs.

Other agencies in the USPHS maintain important programs related to FAS, but these programs have much less emphasis on research. The Indian Health Service, the Health Resources and Services Administration (HRSA), and the Substance Abuse and Mental Health Services Administration (SAMHSA) fund services or demonstration projects directly or indirectly related to FAS. At this time, no agency has been able to support research on the clinical aspects of FAS, on the medical treatment of children with FAS, or on the education and remediation of these children.

A notable USPHS program is the Pregnant and Postpartum Women and Their Infants (PPWI) initiative. This program was authorized by the Anti-Drug Abuse Act, passed by Congress in 1988. The demonstration grant program focuses on the development of innovative, community-based models of drug prevention, education, and treatment, targeting pregnant and postpartum women and their infants (National Center for Education in Maternal and Child Health, 1993). The program is funded jointly by the Center for Substance Abuse Prevention (CSAP) of SAMHSA and the Maternal and Child Health Bureau of HRSA. It has funded 147 demonstration projects. The most common drug addressed was cocaine, followed by alcohol and polydrug use. Because demonstration projects are rigorously evaluated only infrequently, the nature, utility, and transferability of their findings are difficult to assess.

The Center for Substance Abuse Treatment (CSAT), a part of SAMHSA, was charged by Congress to support grants for residential and outpatient substance abuse treatment for pregnant and postpartum women and their infants (information provided to the committee). CSAT funded 31 residential projects in 20 states in the PPWI program and 34 projects in 24 states in its Residential Treatment for Women and Their Children program. The five treatment programs that serve Native American women include comprehensive services specific to FAS. In addition, CSAT has other activities, such as its Treatment Improvement Protocols, relevant to FAS, but the abuse substance of focus is usually cocaine or opiates, not alcohol.

CONGRESSIONAL INTEREST

In recognition of the seriousness of this problem, which affects both the health and the societal functioning of many Americans, several times in the past few years, members of Congress have introduced legislation related to FAS (see Table 1-2). The bills have focused largely on creating an interagency task force on FAS and increasing resources for prevention programs and prevention research. These bills, with one exception, have never been passed. The U.S. Congress mandated in Section 705 of Public Law 102-321, the ADAMHA Reorganization Act, that the Institute of Medicine (IOM) of the National Academy of Sciences conduct a study of FAS and related birth defects. The National Institute

TABLE 1-2 Congressional Bills Related to Fetal Alcohol Syndrome (FAS) or Women and Alcohol

Bill No. and Date Introduced	Bill Name	Major Sponsor	Overview
H.R. 1322 3/7/91	Comprehensive Indian Fetal Alcohol Syndrome Prevention and Treatment Act	Campbell (D-CO)	Authorize services for the prevention, intervention, treatment and aftercare of American Indian and Alaskan Native children and their families at risk for FAS and fetal alcohol effect (FAE). Authorization of grants to Native American tribes for training, prevention, and intervention programs. Convening of FAS/FAE task force including federal representation and representation from Native American tribes. Would have authorized $10 million annually for FY 1993-1995 and $15 million annually for FY 1996-2000.
S. 923 5/7/93	Comprehensive Fetal Alcohol Syndrome Prevention Act	Daschle (D-SD)	Expand resources for basic and applied epidemiological research related to FAS/FAE. Establish programs to coordinate and support national, state, and community-based public awareness, prevention, and educational programs on FAS/FAE. Establish and facilitate a national surveillance program to monitor the incidence of FAS/FAE and the effectiveness of prevention programs. Establish a task force to foster coordination among federal agencies that conduct FAS/FAE research, prevention, and treatment.
H.R. 3569 11/19/93	Women and Alcohol Research Equity Act of 1993	Morella (R-MD)	Provide for an increase in the amount of federal funds expended to conduct research on alcohol abuse and alcoholism among women. Would have authorized up to $23,250,000 to enable NIAAA to increase such research.

Bill/Date	Title	Sponsor	Description
H.R. 3783 2/2/94	Comprehensive Fetal Alcohol Syndrome Prevention Act	Richardson (D-NM)	Establish a comprehensive program to help prevent FAS and FAE and to coordinate federal efforts to prevent FAS and FAE. CDC to coordinate and support applied epidemiologic research on FAS and FAE. NIAAA to conduct and support basic research targeted to developing data to improve prevention and treatment of FAS and FAE. Develop a plan to disseminate diagnostic criteria to health care and social services providers. Establish an inter-agency task force on FAS and FAE. SAMHSA to support, conduct, and evaluate training programs for professionals; and prevention and education programs for the public.
S 170 1/5/95	Comprehensive Fetal Alcohol Syndrome Prevention Act	Daschle (D-SD)	Establish interagency task force on FAS and FAE. Organize a program of basic research on services and effective prevention, treatment and intervention for pregnant alcohol-dependent women and those with FAS or FAE [Originally introduced as S. 1821 in previous session but died in committee.]
H.R. 1649 5/16/95	Comprehensive Fetal Alcohol Syndrome Prevention Act	Richardson (D-SD)	Establish a program for the conduct and support of research and training and the dissemination of health information about the cause, diagnosis, prevention and treatment of FAS and related conditions. Establish an Interagency Coordinating Committee on Fetal Alcohol Syndrome. Develop uniform criteria for the collection and reporting of data on FAS and related conditions.

NOTE: CDC = Centers for Disease Control and Prevention; NIAAA = National Institute on Alcohol Abuse and Alcoholism; and SAMHSA = Substance Abuse and Mental Health Services Administration.

on Alcohol Abuse and Alcoholism of the National Institutes of Health funded the project. This report is in response to that mandate.

The Committee to Study Fetal Alcohol Syndrome was convened in mid-1994. Committee expertise included pediatrics, developmental psychology and neurology, obstetrics, nosology, teratology, epidemiology, sociology, substance abuse prevention and treatment, and psychiatry. The charge to the committee was to improve the understanding of available research knowledge and experience on:

- tools and approaches for diagnosing FAS and related disorders,
- the prevalence of FAS and related disorders in the general population of the United States,
- the effectiveness of surveillance systems, and
- the availability and effectiveness of prevention and treatment programs for these conditions.

As part of its work, the committee assessed and reviewed U.S. Department of Health and Human Services agency research on the topic and provided guidance for the future.

THE COMMITTEE'S FOCUS AND PROCESS

The committee understood its charge to focus on the effects of exposure to large amounts of alcohol, that is, on FAS and what had historically been called fetal alcohol effects (FAE). The committee studied data on the relation between low or moderate levels of prenatal alcohol exposure and more subtle psychologic, educational, developmental, and behavioral abnormalities associated with such exposure, but given the currently available data it was unable to conclude that these subtle abnormalities do or do not represent a distinct clinical entity. Thus, the committee concluded that it was inappropriate to develop diagnostic criteria or establish incidence or prevalence estimates for this putative condition. However, some discussion of these data is warranted.

Large prospective studies conducted in several U.S. cities, which are described more fully in other sections of this report, have found statistical associations between low to moderate levels of prenatal alcohol exposure (levels not documented or believed to cause FAS) and effects on a variety of behavioral, educational, and psychological tests. These statistical associations are typically weak and the estimated average effects are usually small, so these results seem to have little clinical significance for individual children (Day et al., 1991; Russell, 1991). The population implications, in theory, can be important for the following reasons. First, one interpretation of these results is that the *small shift in the average* behavioral, educational, and psychological scores in children prenatally exposed to low levels of alcohol theoretically may translate into increases in the number of children below low performance thresholds and decreases in the number of children above high thresholds. Second, these weak population results could also suggest that prenatal exposure to low levels of alcohol occasionally but only *rarely* lead to behavioral, educational, and psychological effects in an individual that do have clinical significance. The clinical significance of small population effects on an individual has not been demonstrated empirically for low-level prenatal alcohol exposure. Finally, these population effects suggest at least a teratologic potential for low-level prenatal alcohol exposure and can provide directions for further research. It is also possible that these effects are spurious, given the difficulties of excluding confounding variables such as stress or nutrition by history alone. Given the current state of our knowledge it is impossible to conclude whether low-level alcohol intake in pregnancy has clinically significant deleterious effects on the individual or not.

The committee is cognizant of the grave concern of many pregnant or preconceptional women and their partners about possible effects of less than heavy consumption of alcohol, and it is also aware that this issue has been and will continue to be debated in the lay press. The committee hopes its report will clarify research questions and design issues for further work in this area. The lack of diagnostic criteria for or more definitive statements regarding possible effects of low to moderate exposure to alcohol should not be interpreted as contradictory to the Surgeon General's warning against drinking alcohol during pregnancy. This will be discussed in more detail in Chapter 7.

The committee did not establish precise lower limits of alcohol exposure associated with significantly increased risk of FAS. Some researchers have attempted such calculations, but the committee felt that it is premature to make such a statement. Maternal factors such as parity, age, history of heavy drinking, and general health status all influence how much alcohol exposure is necessary for FAS. The level of alcohol exposure is generally very high and likely found in only a small percentage of women who drink while pregnant. Recent data suggest that although approximately 40 percent of all women in the United States are abstinent (Wilsnack et al., 1994), approximately 14 percent of women consume 6 or more drinks at least occasionally when they drink (Wilsnack et al., 1994) and approximately 4 percent of women have alcohol abuse or alcohol dependence problems (Grant et al., 1994).

The committee did not establish an incidence or prevalence rate for FAS in the general U.S. population. Rather, the committee reviewed estimates from the scientific literature. Rates in several of the most complete studies are similar—on the order of 0.5 to 3 cases per 1,000 births. The difficulties in determining the extent of the problem are discussed in this report.

Clinical experience has accumulated with helping pregnant alcoholic women to decrease their drinking and with helping children with FAS to learn and perform more like unaffected children (Kleinfeld and Wescott, 1993). However, most of this rich clinical literature derives from anecdote and uncontrolled projects. As such, it is difficult to distinguish what treatments of either the mother or the child are effective and should be implemented on a larger scale— a potentially expensive endeavor. Therefore, the committee has focused its efforts on reviewing and commenting on the knowledge and experience base that derives from research. As such, the report focuses on NIAAA and CDC. The committee felt it more important to discuss gaps in the knowledge base about FAS and to indicate possible directions for new research endeavors that may ultimately lead to the prevention of what some call the only 100 percent preventable birth defect.

The committee met four times for a total of 10 days, reviewed the published literature, and requested and analyzed information from researchers in the field and from relevant USPHS agencies regarding past and future research efforts in this area. Such information included but was not limited to program budgets and grant and contract abstracts. These were provided by NIAAA and CDC. A major source of information about past work in the area is the published literature. For example, most of the published research using animal models of FAS has been funded by NIAAA. Likewise, CDC-funded work on FAS surveillance is published in Morbidity and Mortality Weekly Reports. Representatives of NIAAA and CDC, who sponsor or conduct most of the USPHS research on FAS, met with the committee at its first meeting, described their programs and subsequently also submitted their vision of their future role in FAS. In addition, much of the published literature on FAS was funded by these agencies and stands as a record of their involvement in the area—many CDC and NIAAA grantees (past and present) were available for consultation by the committee. Several state FAS programs, many of which have some CDC funding, also sent in materials about their programs.   Much has been written recently about FAS and related disorders. The Secretary of Health and Human Services submits a special report to Congress every three years on the current state of knowledge about alcohol and health (U.S. Department of Health and Human Services, 1993). These reports contain superlative reviews of the current state of the published scientific literature on FAS research. In addition, during the course of its deliberations, the committee had access to a volume of papers, published by NIAAA (1994), on FAS. Rather than duplicate those efforts, the committee briefly reviews the established scientific literature on FAS where needed and the reader is referred to the sources cited above for background or more extensive information. As such, this report is relatively brief.

The experimental literature regarding FAS can be complicated. Research in teratology can be intricate and complex. The report lays out some of the basic principles of teratology and how they apply to the study of alcohol and FAS, particularly with animal models, in Chapter 2. Studies in animals are compelling in the context of the human situation. FAS is important because it is a condition caused by human behavior that affects human health and behavior. The committee has tried to paint a portrait of the wide-ranging human dilemmas involving

FAS through vignettes in Chapter 3. These are intended to illustrate the scope and impact of FAS more fully than any individual chapter could. To address the many issues raised by FAS, such as ascertaining its prevalence and assessing therapeutic or prevention interventions, it is essential to maintain well-defined diagnostic criteria. In Chapter 4, the committee has elaborated the principles of setting diagnostic criteria and has presented revised FAS diagnostic criteria, which it recommends for general usage. The diagnostic criteria are essential for surveillance and epidemiologic research on FAS. Current challenges in epidemiology and surveillance of FAS are discussed in Chapter 5. Chapter 6 provides an overview of the epidemiology of women's drinking, an understanding of which is crucial for FAS prevention efforts. Chapter 7 discusses FAS prevention, including treatment for maternal alcohol abuse, while Chapter 8 lays the foundation for research in treatment of the child and the adult with FAS. Chapter 9 consists of a brief summary statement and recommendation concerning the integrative nature of FAS diagnosis, surveillance, prevention, and treatment, and how that impacts on research and treatment challenges.

SOME IMPORTANT DEFINITIONS

Before going further, some clarification of terms is warranted. Several terms are used in this report to refer to drinking patterns and problems. The terms used here are intended to be consistent in spirit with an earlier IOM report *Broadening the Base of Treatment for Alcohol Problems* (IOM, 1990), particularly in their emphasis on the heterogeneity of alcohol problems, the course of alcohol use disorders, patterns of consumption, and etiology. In this schema, alcohol consumption is seen as ranging from none to light to moderate to heavy. Alcohol-related problems (e.g., medical, legal, social, psychological) also range from none to mild to moderate to severe. Research has pointed to a positive correlation between level of alcohol consumption and level of alcohol problems, with the most severe problems generally seen at the highest levels of drinking. This relationship is, however, variable across individuals; that is, in some cases, severe problems can be seen at comparatively moderate levels of drinking.

The fourth edition of the American Psychiatric Association's Diagnostic and Statistical Manual (DSM-IV; 1994) defines alcohol use disorders as alcohol dependence and alcohol abuse. In general, these terms refer to maladaptive patterns of drinking and consequences which constitute a syndrome, usually associated with moderate to heavy alcohol consumption and moderate to severe alcohol-related problems (Edwards et al., 1981; IOM, 1990). In DSM-IV, alcohol dependence is diagnosed when the individual meets three or more of the following seven criteria in a 12-month period: (1) tolerance; (2) withdrawal; (3) drinking in larger amounts or over a longer period than intended; (4) persistent desire or unsuccessful efforts to cut down on drinking; (5) a great deal of time spent drinking or recovering from alcohol effects; (6) declining involvement in social, occupational, or recreational activities because of alcohol use; and (7) use of alcohol despite knowledge of a persistent or recurrent physical or psychological problem caused or exacerbated by that use.

Alcohol abuse is a less severe syndrome characterized by significant adverse consequences associated with alcohol use and is diagnosed when at least one of the following four criteria is met recurrently during a 12-month period: (1) failure to fulfill major role obligations because of alcohol use; (2) recurrent alcohol use in situations when it is physically hazardous; (3) recurrent alcohol-related legal problems; or (4) continued use despite social or interpersonal problems. In addition, the symptoms have never met the criteria for alcohol dependence (American Psychiatric Association, 1994). Alcohol abuse and alcohol dependence have fairly specific meaning in DSM-IV. However, these terms are frequently used as umbrella terms for maladaptive patterns of alcohol use.

In this report on FAS, the committee has chosen to use alcohol abuse as an umbrella term to indicate heavy drinking, including binge drinking, that is risky for the given individual circumstances. If it is clear that a strict DSM-IV diagnosis is intended, it will be so noted. Similar conventions will be used for substance abuse, which is treated very similarly in DSM-IV (American Psychiatric Association, 1994). DSM-IV does not define the term alcoholic, but the National Council on Alcoholism and Drug Dependence does (Morse et al., 1992). Alcoholism, too, is used but only occasionally in this report. It should be noted that there are no specific levels of consumption associated with alcohol abuse, either as used in DSM-IV or as an umbrella term in this report. Survey data from 1992 show that approximately 4 percent of all women and approximately 4 percent of women between the ages of 30 and 44 years of age could be considered to satisfy the DSM-IV criteria for alcohol abuse and alcohol dependence (Grant et al., 1994).

As described in the report, the relation between levels and patterns of drinking during pregnancy and the risk of delivering an infant with FAS is complex. In this report, terms such as "heavy drinking" and "heavier drinking" are used to refer to levels of drinking associated with the highest risk for delivering an infant with FAS. "Binge drinking" is used to refer to a pattern of episodic heavy drinking, which is also associated with higher risk for FAS. Terms such as "risk drinking," or "moderate drinking" are used to indicate lower levels of drinking, usually not associated with FAS, but which may be associated with alcohol-related effects in infants.

It is important to note that definitions of these terms have varied across studies, settings, and samples. In particular, operational definitions of terms used to describe the level and pattern of drinking in studies of *pregnant* women frequently have not corresponded to definitions for *women in general*, which in turn often do not correspond to definitions for *men*. For example, a prospective study of the effects of prenatal alcohol exposure defines heavy drinking as an average of one or more drinks per day (Day et al., 1989); a seminal FAS prevention intervention project defined heavy drinking as five or six drinks on some occasions and at least 45 drinks per month (Rosett et al., 1981); large-scale surveys of drinking in women usually define heavy drinking as two or more standard drinks per day, where a standard drink contains approximately 0.5 ounce of absolute alcohol); some clinical research projects define heavy drinking in women as four or more drinks per day (Wilsnack et al., 1994), which differs from parallel definitions of heavy drinking in men (six or more standard drinks per day). The lack of consistency in terms regarding level of alcohol consumption across studies has led to confusion regarding the relationship between specific levels of drinking and risk for fetal alcohol syndrome and alcohol-related effects (see Abel and Kruger, 1995 for a review of this problem). The committee defines the relevant history for diagnosis of FAS (see Chapter 4) as one of a pattern of excessive intake characterized by substantial, regular intake or heavy episodic drinking. Evidence of this pattern may include: frequent episodes of intoxication, development of tolerance or withdrawal, social problems related to drinking, legal problems related to drinking, engaging in physically hazardous behavior while drinking, or alcohol-related medical problems such as hepatic disease.

REFERENCES

Abel EL, Kruger ML. Hon v. Stroh Brewery Co.: What do we mean by "moderate" and "heavy" drinking? Alcoholism: Clinical and Experimental Research 1995; 19:1024-31.

Abel EL, Sokol RJ. Incidence of fetal alcohol syndrome and economic impact of FAS-related anomalies. Drug and Alcohol Dependence 1987; 19:51-70.

Abel EL, Sokol RJ. A revised conservative estimate of the incidence of FAS and its economic impact. Alcoholism: Clinical and Experimental Research 1991; 15:514-524.

American Psychiatric Association. Diagnostic and Statistical Manual of Mental Disorders: 4th Edition. Washington, DC: American Psychiatric Association, 1994.

Bloss G. The economic cost of FAS. Alcohol Health & Research World 1994; 18:53-54.

Blume SB. Women and Alcohol: Issues in Social Policy in Alcohol and Gender. R. W. Wilsnack and S. C. Wilsnack (eds.). New Brunswick, New Jersey: Rutgers University Center of Alcohol Studies, in press.

Chavkin W. Drug Addiction and Pregnancy: Policy crossroads. American Journal of Public Health 1990; 80:483-487.

Clarren SK, Smith DW. The fetal alcohol syndrome. New England Journal of Medicine 1978; 298; 1063-1067.

Day NL, Jasperse D, Richardson G, Robles N, Sambamoorthis U, Taylor P et al. Prenatal exposure to alcohol: Effect on infant growth and morphologic characteristics. Pediatrics 1989; 84:536-541.

Day NL, Robles N, Richardson G, Geva D, Taylor P, Scher M et al. The effects of prenatal alcohol use in the growth of children at three years of age. Alcoholism: Clinical and Experimental Research 1991; 15:67-71.

Edwards G, Arif A, Hodgson R. Nomenclature and classification of drug- and alcohol-related problems: A WHO memorandum. Bulletin of the World Health Organization 1981; 59:225-242.

Grant BF, Harford RC, Dawson DA, Chou P, Dufour M, Pickering R. Epidemiologic Bulletin No. 35: Prevalence of DSM-IV alcohol abuse and dependence: United States, 1992. Alcohol Health & Research World 1994; 18:243-248.

Harwood HJ, Napolitano DM. Economic implications of the fetal alcohol syndrome. Alcohol Health & Research World 1985; 10:38-43.

Institute of Medicine. Broadening the Base of Treatment of Alcohol Problems. Washington, DC: National Academy Press, 1990.

Jones KL, Smith DW. Recognition of the fetal alcohol syndrome in early infancy. Lancet 1973; 2:999-1001.

Jones KL, Smith DW, Ulleland CH, Streissguth AP. Pattern of malformation in offspring of chronic alcohol mothers. Lancet 1973; 1:1267-1271.

Kleinfeld J, Wescott S. Fantastic Antone Succeeds!: Experiences in educating children with fetal alcohol syndrome. Fairbanks: University of Alaska Press, 1993.

Lemoine P, Harouseau H, Borteryu JT, Menuet JC. Les enfants des parents alcooliques: Anomalies observees apropos de 127 cas. Ouest Medical 1968; 21:476-482.

Morse RM, Flavin DK. The Definition of Alcoholism. Journal of the American Medical Association 1992; 268:1012-1014.

National Center for Education in Maternal and Child Health. Prevention of Perinatal Substance Use: Pregnant and Postpartum Women and Their Infants Demonstration Grant Program—Abstracts of Active Projects Fiscal Year 1993. Arlington, VA: National Center for Education in Maternal and Child Health. 1993.

National Institute on Alcohol Abuse and Alcoholism. Alcohol Health & Research World—[Special Focus: Alcohol-Related Birth Defects]. Dianne M. Welsh (ed.). 18. 1994.

National Institute on Drug Abuse. NIDA survey examines extent of women's drug use during pregnancy. NIDA Media Advisory. Rockville, MD: NIDA, 1994.

Robinson GC, Conry JL, Conry RF. Clinical profile and prevalence of fetal alcohol syndrome in an isolated community in British Columbia. Canadian Medical Association Journal 1987; 137:203-207.

Rosett HL, Weiner L, Edelin KC. Strategies for prevention of fetal alcohol effects. Obstetrics and Gynecology 1981; 57:1-7.

Russell M. Clinical implications of recent research on the fetal alcohol syndrome. Bulletin of the New York Academy of Medicine 1991; 67:207-222.

U.S. Department of Health and Human Services. Alcohol and Health [Eighth Special Report to the U.S. Congress]. DC: U.S. Department of Health and Human Services, 1993.

U.S. Department of Health and Human Services. NIH Data Book—1993. Bethesda, Maryland: National Institutes of Health, 1993.

U.S. Department of Health and Human Services. Healthy People 2000. Rockville, Maryland: U.S. Department of Health and Human Services, 1991.

U.S. Public Health Service. Surgeon General's Advisory on Alcohol and Pregnancy. Federal Drug Administration Bulletin 1981; 11:9-10.

Wilsnack SC, Wilsnack RW, Hiller-Sturmhofel S. How women drink: Epidemiology of women's drinking and problem drinking. Alcohol Health & Research World 1994; 18:173-181.

2

Issues in Research on Fetal Drug Effects

Alcohol is one of a number of chemically diverse compounds currently recognized to be toxic to the developing central nervous system (CNS) of humans. The neurotoxic properties of these compounds have generally been confirmed in animal studies. Based on their effects, these agents can be divided into two classes of neurotoxicants: some are teratogens in that they produce CNS malformations with associated neurobehavioral dysfunction (e.g., alcohol, methylmercury), whereas others produce neurobehavioral dysfunction in the absence of CNS malformations (e.g., lead, polychlorinated biphenyls). The agents in Table 2-1 are presented here in order to put alcohol in the context of other developmental toxic agents and the way these agents can injure the developing CNS, both pre- and postnatally.

Alcohol is a member of one broad category of teratogenic chemicals; this category also includes other substances of abuse (nicotine), pharmacologic agents (phenytoin or retinoic acid), and environmental toxicants (lead, mercury). Other teratogens can be categorized as either physical agents, such as ionizing radiation or hyperthermia; infectious agents, such as rubella virus; and factors related to maternal health and nutrition, such as malnutrition or maternal hyperglycemia secondary to diabetes. Although the effects of exposure to many of these compounds are well described, the mechanisms of action are not. Teratogens differ in their periods of susceptibility, the duration of exposure required to cause adverse fetal outcome, and the manifestations of the insult. A few examples of well-known teratogens are provided below, but this discussion is not exhaustive. This

33

TABLE 2-1 Neurobehavioral Outcome of Prenatal Exposure in Humans or Animals

	Alcohol	Methylmercury	Ionizing Radiation	Phenytoin	PCBs	Lead	Opioids	Marijuana	Tobacco
Gross neuropathology	Pos., NDR	Pos., DR	Pos., DR	—	—	NE	NE	NE	NE
Mental retardation	Pos., DR	Pos., DR	Pos., DR	NE	?	NE	NE	NE	NE
Reduced IQ scores	Pos., DR	Pos., DR	Pos., DR	Pos., NDR	Pos., NDR	Pos., DR	NE	?	Pos., DR
Hyperactivity	Pos., DR	—		—	Pos., NDR	?	NE	NE	Pos., DR
Attention deficit	Pos., DR	—	—	Pos., NDR	—	?	?	Pos., NDR	Pos., NDR
Developmental delays	Pos., DR	Pos., DR	—	—	Pos., DR	—	?	Pos., NDR	Pos., DR
Gait abnormality	Pos., DR	Pos., DR	—	—	NE	NE	NE	NE	NE
Fine/gross coordination	Pos., DR	—	—	—	Pos., DR	?	?	NE	NE
Sensory deficits	Pos., DR	Pos., DR	—	—	NE	Pos., NDR	NE	NE	Pos., DR
Neonatal withdrawal	Pos., NDR	—	—	—	—	—	Pos., DR	?	Pos., DR

NOTE: Pos., DR = Positive findings, dose-related; Pos., NDR = positive findings, non-dose-related; NE = no effects; ? = suspected, some reports; and — = not tested, unknown.

chapter is intended to highlight issues of concern in FAS; the interested reviewer is referred to the published literature for more detail on the other teratogens.

Alcohol is a recognized human teratogen that produces fetal alcohol syndrome (FAS) and a variety of other alcohol-related effects in children exposed during prenatal life. Of all the substances of abuse, including heroin, cocaine, and marijuana, alcohol produces by far the most serious neurobehavioral effects in the fetus.

The teratogenicity of **X-irradiation** has been known since the early part of this century, and it is well-established that the developing CNS is particularly sensitive to irradiation-induced injury. Population-based studies of the effects of in utero exposure in Hiroshima and Nagasaki have indicated a risk of mental retardation based on gestational age at the time of exposure. What would become known as "fetal Minamata disease" results from maternal ingestion of **methylmercury**-contaminated food. Mercury pollutants contained in wastewater and discharged from a chemical plant in Minamata, Japan, accumulated in fish and shellfish, an important staple of the local inhabitants' diet. Even though most of the exposed mothers did not show symptoms of mercury poisoning, exposure of the fetus during gestation months 6-8 produced widespread neuropathological effects in the cerebrum and cerebellum (Burbacher et al., 1990).

Of all the neurotoxicants, **lead** has been the most extensively studied and is viewed as a serious pediatric public health problem. Pregnant women and children living in major urban centers where soil and dust become contaminated with lead-based paint are at risk for undue exposure. Increases in blood levels of lead are known to occur in children as soon as they begin to crawl and to place contaminated hands and toys in their mouth. Neurobehavioral processes of cognition, learning, and behavior are all known to be adversely affected in exposed children (Davis et al., 1990). The **polychlorinated biphenyls** (PCBs), first introduced in the 1930s, are a group of synthetic hydrocarbons that had widespread commercial use as electrical insulating fluid, in heat exchangers, plastics, transformers, capacitors, and carbonless copy paper. As a result of their largely uncontrolled disposal and exceptional persistence, they became a major environmental pollutant in the air, water, and soil of industrialized countries. Children prenatally exposed to PCBs show neurobehavioral effects on cognition, learning, and behavior (Tilson et al., 1990).

Diphenylhydantoin (DPH, phenytoin) is one of several prescription medications, used often in combination, to treat seizures associated with epilepsy. DPH has been implicated as a human teratogen. Although only a relatively small number of children prenatally exposed to DPH have been assessed for neurobehavioral effects, results tentatively suggest a reduction in IQ scores (Adams et al., 1990).

The opiates **heroin** and **methadone** are not teratogenic, and effects on the developing CNS appear to be mediated by the opioid receptors. Neonates show acute but transitory symptoms of neonatal withdrawal, a physiological state characterized by CNS irritability. The symptoms, though life-threatening when severe, are timelimited and resolve in several weeks to months (Hutchings, 1990). Although there have been reports of mild neonatal withdrawal following maternal use of **marijuana**, neurobehavioral deficits are not evident between 6 months and 2 years of age. Beginning at 3 years of age, however, there have been reports of reduced IQ scores (Day et al., 1994), attention deficit (Fried et al., 1992), and developmental delay (Fried, 1993). **Cigarette smoking** during pregnancy is associated with dose-related effects on withdrawal (i.e., increased tremors), reduced IQ scores, developmental delay, and poor auditory responsiveness; several reports have linked maternal smoking with hyperactivity and impaired attention (Fried, 1994). Prenatal exposure to tobacco is clearly linked to low birth weight. Although reports from the mid 1980s suggested that the use of **cocaine** during pregnancy increased the risk of genitourinary tract malformations, abruptio placenta, intrauterine growth retardation, sudden infant death syndrome as well as a number of postnatal neurobehavioral deficits, subsequent reports largely failed to replicate these initial observations (see Hutchings, 1993 and accompanying commentaries). A major problem in interpreting the results of virtually all of the studies that reported these adverse effects is the extent to which the outcomes attributed to cocaine resulted from concurrent abuse of alcohol, cigarettes, and other illicit substances. Ongoing prospective studies that control for these and other confounding variables are expected to yield more interpretable results.

As noted above, alcohol is a potent teratogen; as with most teratogens, there is considerable variation in the extent and severity of prenatal effects in exposed offspring, and that some but not all deficits appear to be attenuated as the offspring matures. For example, a case series of adolescents with FAS show less striking facial dysmorphia and normal weight in some, particularly adolescent females (Streissguth et al., 1985). There are no data suggesting that cognitive deficits ameliorate. Identification of risk factors to explain differences in susceptibility to and expression of alcohol teratogenesis has therefore become an important area of investigation for both basic and clinical researchers. The following sections discuss the contribution of basic research to our understanding of teratology and the potential risk factors that modulate outcomes in fetal alcohol-exposed offspring. This chapter focuses on data from animal models that are relevant to difficult or unanswered issues in clinical FAS research. Chapters 4 and 8 contain discussion relevant to the clinical teratology of alcohol exposure.

PRINCIPLES OF TERATOLOGY AND DEVELOPMENTAL TOXICOLOGY

Wilson (1973) set forth several organizing principles that specify the relationship of environmental agents to adverse outcome: (1) developmental stage; (2) species susceptibility and genotype; and (3) dose-response. Schardein (1985) has succinctly characterized these factors as they relate to teratology by paraphrasing a well-known axiom of Karnofsky (1965); a version modified to include the broader domain of developmental toxicology would be as follows: "A toxic response in developing organisms depends upon the administration of a specific treatment or a particular dose to a genetically susceptible species when the offspring are in a susceptible stage of development." In this section, we extend these basic principles of teratology originally set forth by Wilson (1973) and elaborated by Schardein (1985) to the domain of prenatal alcohol exposure and include the variable of postnatal environment or experience, which is now known to influence developmental outcome.

SUSCEPTIBLE STAGES OF DEVELOPMENT

It is convenient to divide **prenatal development** into three periods: the predifferentiation period, the period of the embryo, and the period of the fetus. The distinction, however, is only conceptual. The conceptus, throughout gestation, is in a continual state of orderly biochemical and structural transition during which new constituents are being formed and spatially rearranged. At any time in the total span of development, these ongoing processes can be subtly deflected, severely perturbed, or abruptly halted, resulting in death or abnormal development. Furthermore, although the effects of exposure during specific stages or "critical periods" of development are probably best documented for the anatomical or dysmorphogenic effects of various teratogenic agents, data on stage-specific effects on growth and functional deficits are increasing, particularly in relation to prenatal alcohol exposure.

The interval between fertilization of the oocyte and its implantation in the endometrium is approximately six days in both rats and humans, and is referred to as the **predifferentiation period**. During this time, the ovum, while remaining relatively undifferentiated, undergoes a series of mitotic divisions, changing from a unicellular zygote to a multicellular blastocyst. Agents that produce malformations later in development are generally thought to be without teratogenic effects during this early period. It appears either that chemicals are toxic to the entire blastocyst, resulting in its death (i.e., spontaneous abortion in humans or resorption in rodents) or that if they are toxic to a limited number of cells, regulative mechanisms result in repair with no apparent damage.

Relatively few studies using animal models have examined the effects of alcohol during the predifferentiation period. An early study reported no adverse effects of alcohol given on gestation day 6 on pregnancy outcome in mice (Lochry et al., 1982). However, in another study (Padmanabhan and Hameed, 1988) it was found that alcohol exposure on gestation days 1-6 did not influence litter size (implantation), but markedly increased prenatal mortality (resorptions) and resulted in increased placental weights, decreased umbilical cord length, and decreased fetal weight at gestation day 15 in surviving litters. Interestingly, malformations (craniofacial, eye, urogenital, limb) were also noted in 80-100 percent of viable fetuses. These somewhat surprising results suggest that very early alcohol exposure, at least in certain mouse strains, may in fact be teratogenic as well as lethal to the embryo.

The period between early germ layer differentiation and the completion of major organ formation (i.e., organogenesis) is referred to as the **period of the embryo**. This phase of development, characterized by the formation of complex, multicellular tissues and organs of diverse origins and functions, begins soon after implantation and, in humans, continues through approximately the eighth week of gestation. During organogenesis, the embryo is maximally susceptible to gross structural malformation if exposed to teratogenic agents. The nature of the defects will depend both on the effects of the agent on embryonic cells and the gestational age at the time of exposure.

In contrast to the predifferentiation period, the effects of acute alcohol exposure on specific days during the embryonic period have been studied fairly extensively. Various mouse strains have been used in these studies, and it is important to note that the results may differ among strains (see section below on "Susceptible Species and Genotype" for discussion of this issue). Teratogenic doses of alcohol induce excessive cell death. Most cell types appear to be vulnerable to alcohol-induced cell death, but neuronal cell populations may be particularly vulnerable. Exposure on gestation days 7 and 8 in mice was shown to result in craniofacial defects similar to those seen in FAS (e.g., micrognathia, low-set ears, short philtrum, cleft palate, cleft lip) (Sulik et al., 1981), as well as brain anomalies (e.g., microcephaly, exencephaly, deficiencies in cerebral hemispheres, striatum, olfactory bulbs, limbic structures, corpus callosum, lateral ventricles) (Sulik et al., 1984; Webster et al., 1980, 1983). In addition, ocular defects (anophthalmia, microphthalmia, corneal and lens anomalies) were associated with acute alcohol exposure on gestation day 7 (Cook et al., 1987; Webster et al., 1983), whereas cardiac (e.g., reduced size of the cardiac tube, abnormalities of the A-V canals, ventricular-septal defects, anomalies of great vessels) (Daft et al., 1986; Webster et al., 1984) and skeletal anomalies (involving vertebrae, sternum, ribs) (Blakely and Scott, 1984; Ciociola and Gautieri, 1988; Padmanabhan and Muawad, 1985; Stuckey and Berry, 1984) were associated with acute exposure on gestation day 8. It was concluded (Kotch and Sulik, 1992) that alcohol teratogenesis and the patterns of malformations induced at times corresponding to late in the third and early in the fourth week postfertilization in the human can be directly correlated to the selective cytotoxic effects of alcohol coupled with the selective vulnerability of the cells at the margin of the anterior neural folds. In contrast, acute alcohol exposure on gestation days 9 and 10 was found to produce urogenital anomalies (hydronephrosis, hydroureter) (Boggan et al., 1989; Gage and Sulik, 1991; Gilliam and Irtenkauf, 1990; Randall et al., 1989) and limb anomalies involving forelimbs (including ectrodactyly, polydactyly, syndactyly) (Gilliam and Irtenkauf, 1990; Kotch et al., 1992; Randall et al., 1989; Webster et

TABLE 2-2 Periods of Susceptibility to Developmental Injuries to the
Nervous System

Developmental injuries to the nervous system have a protracted period of susceptibility that
extends beyond organogenesis. For the central nervous system these include the following
events:

1. Neurogenesis
2. Neuronal differentiation and migration
3. Arborization and synaptogenesis
4. Functional synaptic organization
5. Myelination
6. Gliogenesis, glial migration, and glial differentiation

SOURCE: Adapted from Vorhees (1989).

al., 1980, 1983). A much lower incidence of malformations was observed when
alcohol exposure was restricted to gestation days 12-14.

The interval from the end of organogenesis until parturition (approximately
weeks 9-40 of human pregnancy, corresponding in rats to approximately gestation day 15 to birth) is referred to as the **period of the fetus**. Toxic exposure
during the fetal period generally does not produce gross structural malformations.
Such exposure can, however, produce histologic changes in tissues, inhibit
growth, and produce subtle damage in the developing CNS (often manifested as
neurobehavioral effects) and other organ systems by interfering with histogen-
esis, synaptogenesis, the formation of myelin, and other biochemical processes
(Table 2-2). Such effects are characterized for alcohol by changes in function or
functional organization and include a number of well-documented clinical entities such as microcolon, islet cell hyperplasia, and ventricular septal hypertrophy.
These processes continue well into the **postnatal period** and, for the human
CNS, into the second year of life.

In mouse models, prenatal alcohol exposure on gestation day 15 or 18 was
shown to result in dose-dependent decreases in fetal body weight, decreased
brain DNA (deoxyribonucleic acid) synthesis, and delayed neonatal reflexive
behaviors (Ciociola and Gautieri, 1988). Gestation days 15-21 in the rat also
appear to be a critical period of vulnerability to alcohol-induced reduction in
hippocampal n-methyl-D-aspartate (NMDA) receptor binding (Savage et al.,
1992). However, in terms of CNS effects in rodents, the early postnatal period
may be the most vulnerable to alcohol-induced damage, as it is equivalent to the
third trimester of gestation in humans. For example, it was shown that alcohol
exposure during either the first half or the last half of gestation had no detectable
effect on the development of specific neurons (mossy fibers) within the hippocampus of rats. In contrast, similar alcohol exposure during the first 10 days
postpartum dramatically altered hippocampal mossy fiber organization (West

and Hamre, 1985). Furthermore, with respect to the cerebellum, it was shown that both the extent and the location of neuron loss (specifically, Purkinje and granule cells) were extremely sensitive to the timing of alcohol exposure during the brain growth spurt (Hamre and West, 1993).

Other studies using rat models have shown that late (days 12-17) but not early (days 5-10) gestation is a sensitive period for growth retardation and for behavioral effects of prenatal alcohol exposure. Mice exposed to relatively low alcohol doses (17 percent alcohol-derived calories) had normal birth weights but showed markedly attenuated growth between 19 and 28 days of age, resulting in a weight reduction for at least 35 days (Middaugh and Boggan, 1991). Mice exposed to 25 percent alcohol-derived calories (which led to peak BAC of approximately 100 mg/dl) did not have normal birth weights. It was suggested that fetal alcohol exposure may compromise the organism's ability to handle the increased demands associated with weaning and accelerated growth. Behaviorally, it was reported that fetal alcohol-exposed mice were slower to respond on high fixed ratio schedules than controls (Middaugh and Gentry, 1992). This compromised function may reflect an adverse effect of fetal alcohol exposure on the development of neuronal systems underlying reward which develop during the latter part of gestation.

SUSCEPTIBLE SPECIES AND GENOTYPE

Different species show a differential susceptibility to developmental toxicants, and within species, susceptibility can vary with genotype. For teratological effects, Kalter (1968) pointed out that both inter- and intraspecies variability may be manifested in several ways: (1) an agent that is teratogenic in some species may have little or no teratogenic effect in another; (2) a teratogen may produce similar defects in various species, but these defects will vary in frequency; and (3) a teratogen may induce certain abnormalities in one species that are entirely different from those induced in another. Other critical factors associated with genotype and species relate to differences in rates of metabolism; qualitative differences in metabolic pathways; and for prenatal studies, differences in placental structure and maternal-fetal pharmacokinetics (e.g., see Nau, 1986).

The majority of studies using rodent models have focused on the period of the embryo, which is the primary period of organogenesis. These studies have shown that some mouse strains appear to be particularly sensitive to the teratogenic effects of both acute and chronic alcohol exposure, whereas other strains appear to be less sensitive to alcohol's teratogenic effects (Cassells et al., 1987; Chernoff, 1977). These differences in susceptibility may occur in relation to the teratogenic effects of alcohol on brain morphology as well as to alcohol's effects on the dysmorphology of a number of organ systems. Furthermore, strains may differ in their sensitivity or resistance to alcohol's teratogenic effects depending on the day of exposure, in the sensitivity of particular organ systems that may occur within a strain, or the rate of metabolism of alcohol.

Several recent studies suggest that differences in alcohol sensitivity among organisms with different genotypes may influence the severity of alcohol's effects on the fetus. Studies in mouse lines selectively bred for differences in the hypnotic effects of acute alcohol administration (long sleep [LS] and short sleep [SS]) reported line differences in fetal growth, dysmorphology, behavioral deficits, and mortality that cannot be explained by differences in maternal weight gain, duration of alcohol exposure, or blood alcohol levels (Gilliam et al., 1987; 1989a,b). Offspring of alcohol-sensitive LS mice were shown to exhibit greater prenatal and postnatal growth retardation, increased skeletal abnormalities, deficits in passive avoidance performance, and increased mortality compared to offspring of alcohol-insensitive SS mice. Differences in the pattern of skeletal abnormalities were also observed, with rib anomalies more common in SS fetuses and anomalies of the sternum more common in LS fetuses. Interestingly, it was shown that alcohol-induced deficits in fetal weight were determined primarily by maternal genetic factors, whereas both maternal and fetal genotype appeared to play a role in determining susceptibility to morphological abnormalities (Gilliam and Irtenkauf, 1990).

An important source of information on genetic influences on the expression of teratologic effects comes from studies of twins. Alcohol seems to be similar to many teratogens, such as thalidomide, diethylstilbestrol (DES), and diphenylhydantoin, in that monozygotic twins are more concordant for outcome of prenatal alcohol exposure than dizygotic twins (Streissguth and Dehaene, 1993). This review of 16 pairs of alcohol-exposed twins reports that all five of the monozygotic twin pairs were concordant for diagnosis and that 7 of the 11 dizygotic twins were concordant for diagnosis. In animal studies, not all of the newborns are equally affected. These data suggest that effects of prenatal exposure to alcohol, like many teratogens, can be modulated by genetic influences.

Together these data suggest that genetic factors may, in fact, represent important determinants in susceptibility to teratogenesis, conferring special sensitivity or resistance to the teratogenic effects of alcohol at particular periods of development. However, no specific genes have been identified to date. Clearly, these data have implications for the variability of defects observed in children exposed to high doses of alcohol prenatally.

DOSE-RESPONSE EFFECTS

Dose-response relationships are among the most critical issues in developmental toxicology, yet they are too often misunderstood, oversimplified, or simply neglected. Because prenatal drug studies involve two mutually interacting biological systems, the maternal and fetoplacental dose-response relationships are exquisitely complex and involve interactive pharmacological and toxic effects in the mother and the offspring. An appreciation of the problem may be developed with a few examples.

Both thalidomide and isotretinoin are examples of compounds that produce gross structural malformations in the offspring at levels that are pharmacologically active in the mother (lowest observable effect level, LOEL) but are below the dose that produces maternal toxicity. Among human teratogens, such potent teratological effects are relatively rare. Both vitamin A and salicylate are examples of teratogens that produce functional effects at a lower dose range and dysmorphology at a higher dose range (for review, see Hutchings, 1983). Below a dose level that is lethal to the embryo, there may be two embryotoxic responses, each with its respective threshold. As dose increases above the "no observable effect level" (NOEL), the first embryotoxic response is an impairment in function (lowest observable adverse effect level, LOAEL), followed by a second threshold after which gross structural malformations are produced. THC (Delta-9-tetrahydrocannabinol), the psychoactive ingredient in marijuana, is an example of a compound that produces fetal lethality or growth retardation in the offspring but only at doses that are highly toxic to the mother (Hutchings et al., 1989). Within the pharmacological range of the compound, and at levels that are not toxic to the mother, there is no embryotoxic response. Embryotoxicity is seen only at levels that produce maternal toxicity. This is one of the most common types of profiles observed in animal studies.

Figure 2-1 presents hypothetical dose-response effects for alcohol in the maternal-fetoplacental unit. These relationships are conceptual and not intended to depict empirically established correlations. The general scheme depicts a maternal dose-response function in the lower bar and an embryonic-fetal dose-response function in the upper bar. Overall, as the maternal dose or intake of alcohol increases from no observable effects to progressively greater levels of intoxication, there is a corresponding increase in adverse effects in the fetus. For both the mother and the embryo/fetus, there may be levels of alcohol exposure that produce pharmacological effects (LOEL) but are below the threshold dose for adverse effects (LOAEL). However, the relationship of maternal to fetal dose response effects is incompletely understood. Although the data strongly support a relationship of chronic high levels of maternal alcohol intake to the full FAS, what remains unclear is whether there is a continuum of dose-response effects ranging from anatomic and behavioral changes at low to moderate maternal doses to full-blown FAS at high maternal doses, or if there are two or more thresholds resulting in degrees of impairment in function and structural malformation. As yet undefined is whether there is a LOEL distinct from the LOAEL for alcohol exposure in the fetus.

Dose-response effects of prenatal alcohol exposure have been demonstrated in numerous animal studies. Definitions of what constitutes "high," "moderate," and "low" doses of alcohol in the animal literature vary. Given the differences in alcohol metabolism between humans and rodents (most commonly used in ani-

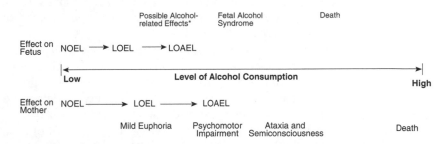

FIGURE 2-1 Maternal/fetal dose-response effects (modified after Hutchings, 1985). *Historically referred to as fetal alcohol effects or alcohol-related birth defects (see Chapter 4). NOEL, no observable effect level; LOEL, lowest observable effect level; LOAEL, lowest observable adverse effect level.

mal models), as well as among species and strains of rodents, levels of alcohol exposure are probably best judged by blood alcohol levels reached rather than quantity or dose of alcohol level administered. Blood alcohol concentrations (BAC) in humans above about 100 mg/dl (0.10 percent) can be considered high; levels of about 50-100 mg/dl can be considered moderate; and levels below about 50 mg/dl can be considered low (U.S. Department of Health and Human Services, 1993). A BAC of 100 mg/dl is considered legal intoxication in most states. A man weighing 150 pounds who consumed two drinks in one hour would have a BAC around 40 mg/dl. Women generally achieve a higher BAC than men at the same level of consumption, even if matched for weight. Peak BAC has been shown in animal models to be more relevant to fetal outcome than the dose administered; this is consonant with clinical experience that binge drinking is risky to the fetus. BACs that are associated with adverse fetal outcomes in rodent models can range from below 50 mg/dl over a period of days to over 400 mg/dl on one day, depending on the outcome examined (Middaugh and Bogan, 1991; Savage et al., 1992; Sulik et al., 1981; West, 1987; West et al., 1990).

In two early studies using mouse models, dose-response effects were observed for malformations induced by prenatal alcohol exposure. Chernoff (1977) found that prenatal alcohol exposure resulted in embryolethality at high doses; cardiac and eyelid dysmorphology at moderate doses; and deficient occiput ossification, neural anomalies, and low fetal weight at low doses. Randall et al. (1977) found dose-response increases for percentage of malformed offspring (anomalies including skeletal, cardiovascular, ophthalmic, abdominal, and urogenital). Similarly, Abel and Dintcheff (1978) reported that postnatal growth deficits in rats increased with increasing alcohol dose. Dose-response effects for behavioral deficits induced by prenatal alcohol exposure have also been reported. For example, linear dose-response functions for spontaneous alternation, reversal learning, and conditioned taste aversion learning tasks were observed for rats exposed to alcohol prenatally. Performance in a passive avoidance task was also found to be directly related to the amount of alcohol consumed by pregnant females (Lochry and Riley, 1980; Riley et al., 1979, 1986).

Alcohol exposure during the early postnatal period (i.e., the third trimester equivalent, reveals similar dose-response effects on both physical and behavioral development. Effects on brain growth during this period of rodent brain growth spurt were particularly marked. Data from West's laboratory (Bonthius and West, 1988; Bonthius et al., 1988) demonstrated that the pattern of alcohol exposure influences the pattern of blood alcohol levels and the severity of brain growth restriction. A particular dose of alcohol administered in multiple feedings over 24 hours has significantly fewer adverse effects than the same dose condensed and administered over a shorter period of time. That is, the more concentrated the pattern of alcohol administration, the higher are the maximum blood alcohol levels achieved and the more severe is the interference with brain growth. Thus, the pattern of alcohol exposure is important because of the resultant blood alcohol concentrations. Increasing doses of alcohol resulted in effects ranging from no significant microcephaly, to decreases in both total brain weight and cerebellar weight, to significant restriction of brain stem weight, to death.

It was also shown that male offspring exhibited greater reduction in brain weight and higher blood alcohol levels than female offspring at a given dose. Thus, males appear more susceptible than females to the adverse effects of alcohol on brain growth (Pierce and West, 1986). Sensorimotor development also appears to be delayed or disrupted with condensed rather than uniform alcohol exposure regimens (Kelly et al., 1987). In addition, deficits in both acquisition and retention of a passive avoidance task were dose related. Together, these data indicate that "bingeing" results in more severe deficits in brain growth, morphology, neuron cell death, sensorimotor development, and behavior than does continuous exposure to the same overall dose of alcohol.

Work from Savage's laboratory suggests that in rats exposure to low to moderate doses of alcohol during the prenatal period may alter certain specific aspects of brain function without inducing gross abnormalities. Prenatal exposure (through a 3.5 percent alcohol liquid diet for varying periods during gestation) resulting in peak maternal blood alcohol levels as low as 40 mg/dl resulted in alterations in hippocampal NMDA receptor binding and in long-term potentiation (Queen et al., 1993; Savage et al., 1992). This level of exposure is significantly less than that required for most alcohol-induced teratogenic effects. In general, the hippocampus, which has an integral role in memory, is particularly sensitive to a number of neurotoxicants, including alcohol. The mechanisms are unclear and may be mediated by alcohol effects on other systems. Changes such as NMDA receptor binding could be one biologic mechanism underlying some of the functional deficits associated with prenatal alcohol exposure.

Data from Clarren and colleagues (Clarren et al., 1988), using a nonhuman primate model, examined the effects of weekly exposure to varying doses of alcohol on specific dysfunctional outcomes. In addition to dose effects, these investigators also examined effects of full gestational exposure (from the first week of gestation) compared to those of delayed gestational exposure (from the fifth week of gestation). It was found that no animal showed all the features of human FAS, although facial dysmorphia, growth deficiency, and CNS dysfunction were found in 16 of the 28 alcohol-exposed animals. Importantly, the data demonstrated that full gestational exposure at doses resulting in blood alcohol levels greater than 140 mg/dl led to significant developmental delays, whereas delayed gestational exposure (exposure to much higher levels of alcohol after gestation week 5) led to animals who were more cognitively intact at 6 months of age. This latter observation was confirmed in follow-up studies in which animals exposed to peak maternal blood alcohol levels of >140 mg/dl once per week in the first six weeks of gestation had the same degree of developmental delay as animals exposed to the same dosages nearly throughout gestation. Thus, measurable teratogenic effects from weekly exposures to alcohol occurred only at intoxicating doses. However, early gestational exposure was more damaging to cognitive function than later—and considerably greater—alcohol exposure. These data are counter-intuitive to current thoughts about nervous system teratology. Although the sample size was small, the data were replicated within the same laboratory. Thus, possible interactive effects of dose of alcohol consumed and susceptible periods of exposure must thus be considered in examining the teratogenic consequences of prenatal alcohol exposure. Interestingly, these investigators have recently shown that modern imaging techniques may be useful in elucidating mechanisms of alcohol teratogenicity. They demonstrated that the choline:creatine ratio in the brain, detected by proton magnetic resonance imaging (MRI), increased significantly with increasing duration of in utero alcohol exposure. These signal alterations occurred in the absence of gross structural brain anomalies (detected by MRI) and were significantly correlated with alcohol-related cognitive and behavioral dysfunction (Astley et al., in press).

INTERVENTION AND PREVENTION

The area of intervention and treatment of children with FAS is still in a relatively young stage. Animal models designed to investigate mechanisms of alcohol teratogenesis and the effects of postnatal and postweaning experiences on developmental outcome may provide insights useful for developing treatment strategies for children with FAS and other alcohol-related birth defects.

A series of studies by Randall and colleagues demonstrated that prostaglandins (PGs) may play a role in the etiology of alcohol-related birth defects. Acute alcohol administration on a single day of pregnancy in mice resulted in decreased fetal weight and increased prenatal mortality and birth defects, particularly kidney and limb defects. Pretreatment with aspirin, which affects prostaglandin metabolism, was found to reduce prenatal mortality and decrease the incidence of birth defects in a dose-dependent manner. Importantly, aspirin dose-dependently inhibited PG levels in uterine and embryonic tissue, and the magnitude of inhibition was positively correlated with the extent to which aspirin reduced the incidence of alcohol-related birth defects (Randall and Anton, 1984; Randall et al., 1991a). Furthermore, the protective effects of aspirin were not related to an effect on maternal blood alcohol levels. Other nonsteroidal anti-inflammatory (NSAI) agents such as ibuprofen and indomethacin were also effective in attenuating alcohol's teratogenic effects but to a lesser extent than aspirin. For example, ibuprofen antagonized the effects of alcohol on fetal growth retardation and the frequency of birth defects, but did not affect prenatal mortality or the number of implantation sites (Randall et al., 1991b). Indomethacin, which does not cross the placenta as readily as aspirin, was found to reduce the number of fetuses with birth defects and appeared to antagonize prenatal mortality, but only at the highest doses (Randall et al., 1987). Clearly, further investigation is needed on the role of prostaglandin in mediating the teratogenic effects of alcohol and on the possible use of PG inhibitors in attenuating alcohol-related birth defects.

A series of studies by Wainwright and colleagues investigated the possibility that adverse effects of fetal alcohol exposure on brain development might be mediated in part by an alcohol-induced reduction of available long-chain polyunsaturated fatty acids to the developing brain (Wainwright et al., 1990a,b). Interestingly, these studies reported that supplementation of the maternal diet with a source of long-chain fatty acids increased maternal weight gain, improved perinatal survival of offspring, increased offspring body weights, and enhanced neurobehavioral development. Furthermore, the fatty acid composition of the maternal diet was found to modulate the effects of prenatal alcohol exposure on the membrane phospholipid composition of the developing brain. Although the magnitude of the effects appears to be small, these data nevertheless suggest the intriguing possibility that alcohol-nutrition interactions may be important in mediating certain critical effects of prenatal alcohol on development.

Both the postnatal and the postweaning rearing environment may also have a critical impact on the developmental outcome of fetal alcohol-exposed offspring. Data from Weinberg et al. (1995) demonstrated that a simple noninvasive manipulation, early postnatal handling, can alter or attenuate some but not all deficits resulting from prenatal alcohol exposure. Handling eliminated deficits in preweaning growth of offspring and performance in a step-down avoidance task, and attenuated the hypothermic response to alcohol challenge as well as the increased adrenocortical response to restraint stress. However, handling had no effect on the corticosterone response to alcohol challenge and did not reduce the more prolonged corticoid elevation during restraint stress observed in alcohol-exposed compared to pair-fed and control animals. Hannigan and coworkers (1993) demonstrated that fetal alcohol-exposed offspring placed in an enriched postweaning environment show an attenuation of gait ataxia and improved performance in a Morris water maze compared with offspring reared in isolation.

Together, the data from these studies clearly have important clinical implications. Data from clinical studies suggest that postnatal environment and experience may significantly influence outcome in terms of both behavioral and cognitive development (Brown et al., 1991; Smith and Coles, 1991). Although one cannot directly extrapolate from findings in animals to the clinical setting, the present data certainly indicate one possible direction for future research on the treatment of children exposed to alcohol prenatally.

A MULTIFACTORIAL MODEL

The data presented above clearly indicate that the teratogenic effects of prenatal alcohol exposure can be influenced by numerous factors, both biological and environmental. The complex nature of these multifactorial influences is illustrated in Figure 2-2. This figure attempts to illustrate the point that the

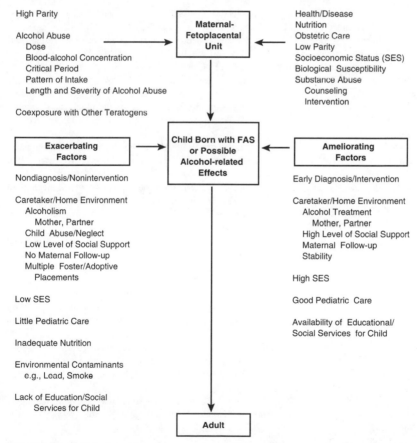

FIGURE 2-2 Theoretical influences on the expression of prenatal alcohol exposure.

expression of adverse alcohol effects in the offspring from birth to adulthood can be influenced by factors that include the critical period during pregnancy when exposure occurs, the pattern and amount of maternal alcohol intake, and a host of biological and environmental variables that can possibly impact both the pre- and the postnatal periods.

The central developmental concepts in the animal research described above provides a framework for understanding the human experience with exposure to alcohol in pregnancy. These concepts include diversity in the degree of injury to fetuses with comparable alcohol exposure, the potential for injury throughout fetal life, a relationship between level of alcohol exposure and degree of injury, and the importance of both biological variables and the postnatal environment in influencing outcome.

REFERENCES

Abel EL, Dintcheff BA. Effects of prenatal alcohol exposure on growth and development in rats. Journal of Pharmacology and Experimental Therapeutics 1978; 207:916-921.

Adams J, Vorhees CV, Middaugh LD. Developmental neurotoxicity of anticonvulsants: Human and animal evidence on phenytoin. Neurotoxicology and Teratology 1990; 12:203-214.

Astley SJ, Weinberger E, Shaw DWW, Richards TL, Clarren SK. Magnetic resonance imaging and spectroscopy in fetal ethanol exposed Macaca nemestrina. Neurotoxicology and Teratology, in press.

Blakely PM, Scott WJ, Jr. Determination of the proximate teratogen of the mouse fetal alcohol syndrome: Teratogenicity of ethanol and acetaldehyde. Toxicology and Applied Pharmacology 1984; 72:355-363.

Boggan WO, Monroe B, Turner WR, Upshur J, Middaugh LD. Effect of prenatal ethanol administration on the urogenital system of mice. Alcoholism: Clinical and Experimental Research 1989; 13:206-208.

Bonthius DJ, Goodlett CR, West JR. Blood alcohol concentration and severity of microencephaly in neonatal rats depend on the pattern of alcohol administration. Alcohol 1988; 5:209-214.

Bonthius DJ, West JR. Blood alcohol concentration and microencephaly: A dose-response study in the neonatal rat. Teratology 1988; 37:223-231.

Brown RT, Coles CD, Smith IE, Platzman KA, Silverstein J, Erickson S et al. Effects of prenatal alcohol exposure at school age. II. Attention and behavior. Neurotoxicology and Teratology 1991; 13:369-376.

Burbacher TM, Rodier PM, Weiss B. Methylmercury developmental neurotoxicity: A comparison of effects in humans and animals. Neurotoxicology and Teratology 1990; 12:191-202.

Cassells B, Wainwright P, Blom K. Hereditary and alcohol-induced brain anomalies: Effects of alcohol on anomalous prenatal development of the corpus callosum and anterior commissure in BALB/c and C57BL/6 mice. Experimental Neurology 1987; 95:587-604.

Chernoff GF. The fetal alcohol syndrome in mice: An animal model. Teratology 1977; 15:223-230.

Ciociola AA, Gautieri RF. Teratogenic and behavioral anomalies induced by acute exposure of mice to ethanol and their possible relation to fetal brain DNA synthesis. Pharmaceutical Research 1988; 5:447-452.

Clarren SK, Astley SJ, Bowden DM. Physical anomalies and developmental delays in nonhuman primate infants exposed to weekly doses of ethanol during gestation. Teratology 1988; 37:561-569.

Cook CS, Nowotny AZ, Sulik KK. Fetal alcohol syndrome: eye malformations in a mouse model. Archives of Ophthalmology 1987; 105:1576-1581.

Daft PA, Johnston MC, Sulik KK. Abnormal heart and great vessel development following acute ethanol exposure in mice. Teratology 1986; 33:93-104.

Davis JM, Otto DA, Weil DE, Grant LD. The comparative developmental neurotoxicity of lead in humans and animals. Neurotoxicology and Teratology 1990; 12:215-229.

Day NL, Richardson G, Goldschmidt L, Robles N, Taylor P, Stoffer M et al. The effect of prenatal marijuana exposure on the cognitive development of offspring at age three. Neurotoxicology and Teratology 1994; 16:169-176.

Fried PA. Clinical implications of smoking: Determining long-term teratogenicity. Maternal Substance Abuse and the Developing Nervous System. I. S. Sagon and T.A. Slotkin (eds.) Orlando, Florida: Academic Press, 1994.

Fried PA. Prenatal exposure to tobacco and marijuana: Effects during pregnancy, infancy and early childhood. Clinical Obstetrics and Gynecology 1993; 36:319 337.

Fried PA, Watkinson B, Gray R. A follow-up study of attentional behavior in 6-year-old children exposed prenatally to marihuana, cigarettes, and alcohol. Neurotoxicology and Teratology 1992; 14:299-311.

Gage JC, Sulik KK. Pathogenesis of ethanol-induced hydronephrosis and hydroureter as demonstrated following in vivo exposure of mouse embryos. Teratology 1991; 44:299-312.

Gilliam DM, Irtenkauf KT. Maternal genetic effects on ethanol teratogenesis and dominance of relative embryonic resistance to malformations. Alcoholism: Clinical and Experimental Research 1990; 14:539-545.

Gilliam DM, Kotch LE, Dudek BC, Riley EP. Ethanol teratogenesis in mice selected for differences in alcohol sensitivity. Alcohol 1989a; 5:513-519.

Gilliam DM, Kotch LE, Dudek BC, Riley EP. Ethanol teratogenesis in selectively bred long-sleep and short-sleep mice: A comparison to inbred C57BL/6J Mice. Alcoholism: Clinical and Experimental Research 1989b; 13:667-672.

Gilliam DM, Stillman S, Dudek BC, Riley EP. Fetal alcohol effects in Long- and Short-Sleep mice:Activity, passive avoidance, and in utero ethanol levels. Neurotoxicology and Teratology 1987; 9:349-357.

Hamre KW, West JR. The effects of the timing of ethanol exposure during the brain growth spurt on the number of cerebellar Purkinje and granule cell nuclear profiles. Alcoholism: Clinical and Experimental Research 1993; 17:610-622.

Hannigan JH, Berman RF, Zajac CS. Environmental enrichment and the behavioral effects of prenatal exposure to alcohol in rats. Neurotoxicology and Teratology 1993; 15:261-266.

Hutchings DE. The puzzle of cocaine's effects following maternal use during pregnancy: Are there reconcilable differences (Open Peer Commentary). Neurotoxicology and Teratology 1993; 15:281-286.

Hutchings DE. Issues of risk assessment: Lessons from the use and abuse of drugs during pregnancy. Neurotoxicology and Teratology 1990; 12:183-189.

Hutchings, DE. Issues of methodology and interpretation in clinical and animal behavioral teratology studies. Neurobehavioral Toxicology and Teratology 1985; 7:639-642.

Hutchings DE. Behavioral teratology: A new frontier in neurobehavioral research. Handbook of Experimental Pharmacology: Teratogenesis and Reproductive Toxicology. E.M. Johnson and D. M. Kochhar (eds.). New York: Springer-Verlag, 1983.

Hutchings DE, Brake SC, Morgan B. Animal studies of prenatal delta-9-tetrahydrocannabinol: Female embryolethality and effects on somatic and brain growth. Annals of the New York Academy of Sciences 1989; 562:133-144.

Kalter H. Teratology of the Central Nervous System. Chicago: University of Chicago Press, 1968.

Karnofsky DA. Drugs as teratogens in animals and man. Annual Review of Pharmacology 1965; 5:447-472.

Kelly SJ, Hulsether SA, West JR. Alterations in sensorimotor development: Relationship to postnatal alcohol exposure. Neurobehavioral Toxicology and Teratology 1987; 9:243-251.

Kotch LE, Dehart DB, Alles AJ, Chernoff N, Sulik KK. Pathogenesis of ethanol-induced limb reduction defects in mice. Teratology 1992; 46:323-332.

Kotch LE, Sulik KK. Experimental Fetal Alcohol Syndrome:Proposed pathogenic basis for a variety of associated facial and brain anomalies. American Journal of Medical Genetics 1992; 44:168-176.

Lochry EA, Randall CL, Goldsmith AA, Sutker PB. Effects of acute alcohol exposure during selected days of gestation in C3H mice. Neurobehavioral Toxicology and Teratology 1982; 5:15-19.

Lockry EA, Riley EP. Retention of passive avoidance and T-maze escape in rats exposed to alcohol prenatally. Neurobehavioral Toxicology 1980; 2:107-115.

Middaugh LD, Boggan WO. Postnatal growth deficits in prenatal ethanol-exposed mice: Characteristics and critical periods. Alcoholism: Clinical and Experimental Research 1991; 15:919-926.

Middaugh LD, Gentry GD. Prenatal ethanol effects on reward efficacy for adult mice are gestation stage specific. Neurotoxicology and Teratology 1992; 14:365-370.

Nau H. Species differences in pharmacokinetics and drug teratogenesis. Environmental Health Perspectives 1986; 70:113-129.

Padmanabhan R, Hameed MS. Effects of acute doses of ethanol administered at preimplantation stages on fetal development in the mouse. Drug and Alcohol Dependence 1988; 22:91-100.

Padmanabhan R, Muawad WMRA. Exencephaly and axial skeletal dysmorphogenesis induced by acute doses of ethanol in mouse fetuses. Drug and Alcohol Dependence 1985; 16:215-227.

Pierce DR, West JR. Alcohol-induced microencephaly during the third trimester equivalent: Relationship to dose and blood alcohol concentration. Alcohol 1986; 3:185-191.

Queen SA, Sanchez CF, Lopez SR, Paxton LL, Savage DD. Dose- and age-dependent effects of prenatal ethanol exposure on hippocampal metabotropic-glutamate receptor-stimulated phosphoinositide hydrolysis. Alcoholism: Clinical and Experimental Research 1993; 17:887-893.

Randall CL, Anton RF. Aspirin reduces alcohol-induced prenatal mortality and malformations in mice. Alcoholism: Clinical and Experimental Research 1984; 8:513-515.

Randall CL, Anton RF, Becker HC, Hale RL, Ekblad U. Aspirin dose-dependency reduces alcohol-induced birth defects and prostaglandin E levels in mice. Teratology 1991a; 44:521-529.

Randall CL, Becker HC, Anton RF. Effect of ibuprofen on alcohol-induced teratogenesis in mice. Alcoholism: Clinical and Experimental Research 1991b; 15:673-677.

Randall CL, Anton RF, Becker HC, White NM. Role of prostaglandins in alcohol teratogenesis. Annals of the New York Academy of Sciences 1989; 562:178-182.

Randall CL, Anton RF, Becker HC. Effect of Indomethacin on alcohol-induced morphological anomalies in mice. Life Sciences 1987; 41:361-369.

Randall CL, Taylor WJ, Walker DW. Ethanol-induced malformations in mice. Alcoholism: Clinical and Experimental Research 1977; 1:219-224.

Riley EP, Baron S, Hannigan JH. Response inhibition deficits following prenatal alcohol exposure: A comparison to the effects of hippocampal lesions in rats. Alcohol and Brain Development. West, J.R. (ed.). New York: Oxford University Press, 1986:71-102.

Riley EP, Lochry EA, Shapiro NR. Lack of response inhibition in rats prenatally exposed to alcohol. Psychopharmacology 1979; 62:47-52.

Savage DD, Queen SA, Sanchez CF, Paxton LL, Mahoney JC, Goodlett CR et al. Prenatal ethanol exposure during the last third of gestation in rat reduced hippocampal NMDA agonist binding site density in 45-day-old offspring. Alcohol 1992; 9:37-41.

Schardein JL. Chemically Induced Birth Defects. New York: Marcel Dekker, Inc., 1985.

Smith IE, Coles CD. Multilevel intervention for prevention of fetal alcohol syndrome and effects of prenatal alcohol exposure. Recent Developments in Alcoholism, Vol. 9. Galanter M., (ed.) New York: Plenum, 1991:165-180.

Streissguth AP, Clarren SK, Jones KL. Natural history of the fetal alcohol syndrome. A 10-year follow-up of eleven patients. Lancet 1985; 2:85-92.

Streissguth AP, Dehaene P. Fetal alcohol syndrome in twins of alcoholic mothers: Concordance of diagnosis and IQ. American Journal of Medical Genetics 1993; 47:857-861.

Stuckey E, Berry CL. The effects of high dose sporadic (binge) alcohol intake in mice. Journal of Pathology 1984; 142:175-180.

Sulik KK, Johnston MC, Webb MA. Fetal alcohol syndrome: Embryogenesis in a mouse model. Science 1981; 214:936-938.

Sulik KK, Lauder JM, Dehart DB. Brain malformations in prenatal mice following acute maternal ethanoladinistration. International Journal of Developmental Neuroscience 1984; 2:203-214.

Tilson HA, Jacobson JL, Rogan WJ. Polychlorinated biphenyls and the developing nervous system: Cross-species comparisons. Neurotoxicology and Teratology 1990; 12:239-248.

U.S. Department of Health and Human Services. Alcohol and Health [Eighth Special Report to the U.S. Congress]. Washington, DC: U.S. Department of Health and Human Services, 1993.

Vorhees CV. Principles of behavioral teratology. Handbook of Behavioral Teratology. E. P. Riley and C. V. Vorhees, (eds.). New York: Plenum Press, 1986.

Wainwright PE, Huang YS, Simmons V, Ward RP, Ward GR, Winfield D et al. Effects of prenatal ethanol and long-chain n-e fatty acid supplementation on development in mice. 2. Fatty acid composition of brain membrane phospholipids. Alcoholism: Clinical and Experimental Research 1990a; 14:413-420.

Wainwright PE, Ward GR, Winfield D, Huang YS, Mills DE, Ward RP et al. Effects of prenatal ethanol and long-chain n-3 fatty acid supplementation on development in mice. 1. Body and brain growth, sensorimotor development, and water T-Maze reversal learning. Alcoholism: Clinical and Experimental Research 1990b; 14:405-412.

Webster WS, Germain MA, Lipson A, Walsh D. Alcohol and congenital heart defects: An experimental study in mice. Cardiovascular Research 1984; 18:335-338.

Webster WS, Walsh DA, McEwen SE, Lipson AH. Some teratogenic properties of ethanol and acetaldehyde in implications for the study of the fetal alcohol syndrome teratology. Teratology 1983; 27:231-243.

Webster WS, Walsh DA, Lipson AH, McEwen SE. Teratogenesis after acute alcohol exposure in inbred and outbred mice. Neurobehavioral Toxicology 1980; 2:227-234.

Weinberg J, Kim CK, Yu W. Early handling can attenuate adverse effects of fetal ethanol exposure. Alcohol 1995, in press.

West JR. Fetal alcohol-induced brain damage and the problem of determining temporal vulnerability: A review. Alcohol and Drug Research 1987; 7:423-441.

West JR, Hamre KM. Effects of alcohol exposure during different periods of development: Changes in hippocampal mossy fibers. Developments in Brain Research 1985; 17:280-284.

West JR, Goodlett CR, Bonthius DJ, Hamre KM, Marcussen BL. Cell population depletion associated with fetal alcohol brain damage: Mechanisms of BAC-dependent cell loss. Alcoholism: Clinical and Experimental Research 1990; 14:813-818.

Wilson JG. Environment and Birth Defects. New York: Academic Press, 1973.

3

Vignettes

In the following pages, several vignettes are presented to describe a variety of experiences that are frequently encountered in the context of prenatal alcohol exposure, particularly its most severe outcome, fetal alcohol syndrome (FAS). The vignettes are based on interviews of cases known to committee members, but many details have been changed to protect the privacy of individuals. The stories are intended to paint a picture of FAS. Each subsequent chapter of the report describes one piece of the fetal alcohol syndrome problem. The best-known case history of FAS in the lay literature is *The Broken Cord*, a moving account of an adoptive father's struggle to understand the serious limitations of his son (Dorris, 1989). The reader is referred to this work for a complete description of a severe case of FAS. Dorris has also written essays describing the lives of his other adopted children who are affected by prenatal alcohol exposure (included in Dorris, 1994). Dorris' works are particularly important for their description of the difficulties parents have in accepting their child's limitations and of problems faced by prenatal alcohol-affected teenagers and adults.

The first three examples in this chapter are case histories of women who have given birth to children whose problems run the gamut from none to possible alcohol-related effects, to FAS. Following these is a case involving brothers, both affected by prenatal alcohol exposure, with a description of the social setting into which they were born. The next vignette describes the outcome of someone with FAS who was raised in a stable and supportive environment. The next case example describes the life of a woman with fetal alcohol syndrome, including the birth of her four children. Finally, a vignette is described that is quite typical of an alcohol-abusing woman's encounter with the health care system. This case history begins with the birth of a child with fetal alcohol syndrome.

These case histories are presented to provide the reader with the real-life context in which significant fetal alcohol exposure often occurs. The reader will note that there are many *similarities* in the maternal histories presented. Some of these similarities include the following: alcohol abuse is usual in the family of birth of women who drink during pregnancy; early experimentation with alcohol is common; first pregnancy often occurs at a very young age; FAS and other levels of alcohol-related damage usually occur in later pregnancies and in the later years of childbearing; child neglect is frequent; unstable domestic relations are common, particularly when a spouse who abuses alcohol is involved; there is a general lack of stable employment and occupational commitment; and low education and unstable living conditions are frequent. Commonly, there is intervention by others with the children after birth to protect them from chaotic home environments.

The reader will also notice many *differences* among these cases. It cannot easily be said that there is only one pattern that leads to the birth of FAS children. Some of the differences illustrated in the cases are in the quantity, frequency, and timing of the drinking that occurs. That is, there are a number of heavy-drinking patterns, from bingeing to chronic consumption, that can produce FAS. Various levels of medical and health problems are experienced by the mothers, very frequently in some and surprisingly absent in others, given the high level of drinking. Frequent contacts with criminal justice and social service agencies occur, but some women, particularly isolated drinkers, tend to escape this problem. Finally, family relationships are highly variable, although frequently not very stable. Many of the consequences of drinking relate to the level of community support and to the social interaction, both within a community and between the community and the pregnant woman who drinks.

Therefore, despite the commonalities outlined above, there is no one pattern or life-style associated with alcohol abuse or with having a baby with FAS. While we must be aware of the common risk factors and patterns of maternal drinking that can lead to FAS and other possible alcohol-related effects, we must also be aware that any of a variety of patterns of alcohol abuse—particularly over an extended period of time in older women of childbearing age—can damage a fetus.

SALLY

Sally was 35 years old. She had been pregnant three times and had borne two boys and a girl. Her second child was diagnosed with FAS while she was pregnant with the third child. This third child has since been diagnosed with FAS as well. Sally had a relatively unremarkable youth, but was 16 years old at the birth of her first child. The other two children were born when she was 28 and 31 years of age. The oldest child lives with his birth father.

Her overall health has been marked by irregular menses and bouts of weight loss. She has seen a physician for hallucinations and an eating disorder. She has also had several episodes of pneumonia. Her psychiatric and physical problems have been attributed by her physician to her alcohol abuse.

Her first experience with alcohol was at age 16, while she was pregnant, and she reports that she began drinking regularly at 17, after her first baby was born. She was not married, and her parents cared for the child as much as she did. During her twenties she drank heavily, sometimes in weekend binges, but at other times she might remain intoxicated for a week or more at a time. She has been in outpatient alcohol treatment once and has attended Alcoholics Anonymous (AA) meetings sporadically over the years. She did not receive treatment for alcohol dependence during her pregnancies. At the time of interview, she was not in treatment and reported that she continued to drink six beers or wine coolers daily, with binges of more than ten drinks at least once a week. She is not at risk for another FAS child because of a recent tubal ligation.

During the pregnancy with her second child, she reported drinking four to six drinks one to two times per week, generally at local parties in bars in the nearby towns, through the first and second trimesters. She stopped drinking completely toward the end of the pregnancy. She had late prenatal care, starting in the third trimester, and was diagnosed with gestational diabetes. None of her friends used drugs other than alcohol, so neither did she during the pregnancy. She worked part-time at home. She did not live with her partner for most of the pregnancy. The infant weighed 5 pounds, 4 ounces at birth. Her drinking patterns during the third pregnancy were similar.

Sally's father is no longer associated with the family because of his alcohol abuse. Her closest friends are heavy drinkers. Her partner during her second and third pregnancies was a heavy binge drinker. She now lives with her three children; makes money infrequently through domestic jobs; and receives Aid for Families with Dependent Children (AFDC), food stamps, and a government housing subsidy. When she is drinking heavily on binges, members of her extended family look after the children.

ANN

Ann was a 34-year-old who had been pregnant five times and had given birth to five children (three girls and two boys). Each of these children weighed less at birth than the previous one. Her youngest child was diagnosed with FAS. She was 33 when this child was born. There is some concern that the other children have problems, but they have not yet been evaluated by a specialist. All of her children were fathered by the same man. She rarely used birth control of any type.

At the time of interview, all of her children lived with her. However, shortly after the interview she was arrested for abandonment of the children and they were put into foster care with their maternal grandmother.

She has a high school diploma and is a self-employed artisan. Her heath status has been generally good, except for pregnancy-induced hypertension during the last three pregnancies. Depression has been a problem that has taken her to a physician. She has had several injuries as a result of domestic violence, including one during the pregnancy with the child diagnosed as FAS. She reports alcohol involvement in these episodes. Her husband, friends, and her father drank heavily. Her mother does not drink, which is true of many women in this particular community, where drinking is more typically a male recreational activity.

Her first experience with alcohol was at age 12; however, she did not start drinking regularly until she was 20. She has received inpatient treatment for alcohol dependence once and outpatient treatment twice. At the time of interview she was not in treatment and reported binges of more than 10 drinks on the weekends. She also reported past use of marijuana.

During the pregnancy with the child diagnosed with FAS, she drank more than 10 beers almost every day until the last few weeks of the pregnancy, at which time she states that she abstained from alcohol use until after the birth. She was married during the time of the pregnancy and reports that her spouse was a heavy drinker on weekends. She states that she used no other drugs during the pregnancy. She had no prenatal care and was seen by a physician only at delivery.

LYDIA

Lydia was a 36-year-old who had been pregnant eight times. She gave birth to five living children, having had one miscarriage and one intrauterine fetal death at 24 weeks. She was pregnant at the time of interview. Her youngest two children were examined for possible FAS. Her first child was born when she was 19 years old; the children suspected to have FAS were born when she was age 30 and 31. She has been married twice and has had several different partners who have fathered her children. Of her five living children, only two live with her. Her parental rights have been terminated for one of the children seen in a special clinic as a suspected FAS case; the child was adopted by Lydia's sister.

Her first experience with alcohol was at age 16, and she began "drinking regularly" at 21 years of age. She occasionally used marijuana. Her only involvement with alcohol treatment was attendance at AA meetings. At the time of interview, she admitted to current use of alcohol, drinking more than 10 beers once per week with occasional heavier binges. Most of her drinking is done in small groups with friends, either at someone's house, or at home alone with a male friend.

She stated that during the pregnancy with her fourth child, she drank 9 to 10 beers three or four times a week through the first, second, and part of the third trimester, and then abstained in the last few weeks of pregnancy. Most of this drinking was done at home, alone, and in secret. She smoked less than one pack of cigarettes a day. She also received early and adequate prenatal care.

This child, a boy, weighed less than 6 pounds at birth and had facial dysmorphology characteristic of FAS, including short palpebral fissures, flat philtrum, hypoplastic midface, and moderate hirsutism. However, at the time of examination (when the boy was 3 years old), his height was at the 35th percentile, and his head circumference was at the 10th percentile; therefore, he was larger than most FAS children at this age. He manifested some developmental delay but, in the absence of growth deficit, did not receive the diagnosis of FAS from a dysmorphologist (although he had previously been diagnosed as having fetal alcohol effects by a pediatrician).

Lydia stated that during the pregnancy with the youngest child (the fifth) she was still consuming a significant amount of alcohol, but drank less often and smaller amounts than during the pregnancy with the older child. She also decreased the amount of alcohol over the entire course of the pregnancy and did not drink at all during the third trimester. She received early and adequate prenatal care. She continued to smoke during this pregnancy. Her partner, who is also the father of her fourth child, was more stable at this time and lived with her during the entire pregnancy. He nevertheless continued to drink heavily during this time, most frequently at home. Neither had steady jobs. The younger child weighed 6 pounds, 2 ounces, at birth. She does not manifest the dysmorphology or other physical features found in the next older child, although she appears to have some developmental problems that are consistent with a possible alcohol-related effect.

Lydia's social history is significant for heavy alcohol use by her siblings and partner. Her father is a recovering alcoholic. She was once arrested for public intoxication, and she has been involved with child protective services for issues of abuse and neglect. They terminated parental rights for the third child, prior to the birth of the fourth child. She has continued to drink during this current pregnancy, but when contacted by the counselor who performed the interview on which this vignette is based, she was sober and had been so for two days. She seemed genuinely aware, at the time of interview, of the importance of eliminating drinking in this pregnancy.

MARK AND JAMES

Mark and James had been in foster care for four months when they were referred for developmental evaluation. Their foster mother found Mark, 18 months, and James, 31 months, unmanageable and was considering requesting their placement in another foster home. Although she and her husband were experienced foster parents and were being supported by an agency that provided case management, medical services, and education for foster parents, they found dealing with the boys' behavior extremely difficult. Neither child showed any evidence of language development. Mark bit people frequently and often attempted to swallow nonfood items as if he were not able to discriminate food from other items (a condition called "pica"). As a result, he would often choke, and his foster mother was afraid that he would asphyxiate. He interacted with objects inappropriately and threw every object after attempting to bite it. James did not seek contact with people and showed no evidence of emotional reactions. He did not respond to social approaches from adults or other children.

Both children showed irregular sleeping habits, refusing to go to sleep at bedtime, and often awoke during the night and left their beds to roam around the house and to play with things in the dark. Both children refused to eat at the table but preferred to steal food from peoples' plates and from the garbage. The boys were constantly in motion, darting from one object to another, and neither child responded to attempts at discipline on the part of their foster parents or other adults.

At this first assessment, neither child could be tested, although it was evident that they were delayed in the development of language, cognitive, and social skills. Both boys also were mildly delayed in achieving fine and gross motor skills. James appeared to be small for his age but in the normal range (20th percentile), while Mark was at the 3rd percentile for head circumference and weight. Mark also had the characteristic facial features associated with fetal alcohol syndrome.

The caseworker who supervised the brothers' care reported that the boys were "crack" babies and, at that time, she and the foster parents attributed their unusual behavior to prenatal cocaine exposure. However, when the mother's medical records were reviewed, she had a long history of alcohol abuse and had been using cocaine only in the last few years. She was 34 at the time James was born and reported that she had been drinking heavily since she was a teenager. She had been hospitalized on several occasions for alcohol-related injuries, and it was noted at the time of Mark's birth that she was experiencing alcoholic gastritis and had evidence of liver damage. She reported drinking about 12 ounces of absolute alcohol per week (24 drinks) during her pregnancy with James and about 20 ounces a week (40 drinks) when pregnant with Mark. She was also noted to be a polydrug user, who reported smoking about a pack of cigarettes a day, using marijuana regularly, and using cocaine several times a week. When Mark was born, a urine screen revealed the presence of cocaine metabolites, which called the family to the attention of county social service agencies. The mother was assigned a caseworker, who eventually recommended that the children be removed from the home due to neglect. Investigation indicated that the children had received virtually no care over the previous year and that James had been scavenging food from the garbage to feed himself and Mark.

It was recommended that the boys be seen again after a year in foster care, since their behavior indicated that both had an attachment disorder due to lack of caregiving and that neither was socialized enough to allow accurate assessment of their abilities. A stable foster home, good nutrition, and referral to an early intervention program were recommended. When the boys came in for the one-year follow-up, their behavior had changed dramatically. The unresponsive, feral children were now unusually quiet and watchful. Both were responsive to social stimuli and could use language. Problems with eating and sleeping patterns were resolved, and both children were toilet trained. Cognitive testing indicated that James was functioning in the "borderline" range intellectually. That is, he had an IQ of about 75 and his adaptive skills were equivalent. Mark, who had noticeable facial dysmorphia at this time, was functioning in the mildly retarded range (i.e., developmental score of less than 70) with equivalent adaptive skills. The boys were noted to be growth retarded as well, with Mark more affected than James. At $2^1/2$, Mark weighed about 20 pounds and looked somewhat frail. During the assessment, he clung anxiously to his foster mother and appeared very wary.

James is now in first grade, and Mark is in kindergarten. Both continue to show the characteristics of fetal alcohol exposure, with Mark, the younger child, more obviously affected. Both are cognitively delayed, show fine and gross motor deficits, and are small and slender. However, both boys also show the emotional problems associated with early neglect and foster care placement, that is, attachment disorder and, as they have gotten older, conduct disorder. James has experienced a number of problems at school and is being recommended for placement in a classroom for children with behavior disorders. His teacher suggested that he be treated for attention-deficit hyperactivity disorder, but comprehensive medical and psychological assessment did not confirm this diagnosis. Instead, his acting out and angry behavior are attributed to his attachment problems. Mark, who is more clearly mentally retarded, has been able to receive special education services and has had fewer behavior problems. Their foster parents, who have four other children in the home, have provided good basic care but have not been able to make the emotional connections with the boys that might have helped them overcome their early attachment difficulties.

PETER

Peter is 25 years old. His mother began drinking when she was 15 years of age and was alcohol dependent by the time of his birth nine years later. His father was a professional with a good income and was able to shield his wife's alcohol problem from public view. The mother attempted alcohol treatment when Peter was a year old and after a relapse became permanently sober when he was a toddler.

Early schooling did not go easily for Peter. Comprehensive educational testing showed that Peter had borderline intelligence (IQ = 72), problems with language usage, significant delays in reading and math even for his level of intelligence, distractibility and hyperactivity. Peter was placed in special classes and provided with tutoring. He was able to make academic progress with this support but continued to have problems in school because of his failure to follow rules. His parents believed that the child was truly unable to understand the rules, but the teachers would not agree. Peter was regularly punished for his behavior and began to show anger and school anxiety. In addition he was not well accepted by other children his own age and was largely isolated. His parents' response to Peter's emotional change was to remove him from the school. After concluding that Peter would face many of the same assumptions about his behavior in other schools, they decided to teach him at home and to develop his peer group through their church. This approach worked reasonably well, but Peter increasingly asked to return to school and started high school in the ninth grade. He found the level of work and the pace of activity simply too high. He dropped out of school in the tenth grade, but his parents were able to help him get a GED.

After leaving school Peter began to have trouble with the police. He was caught shoplifting on several occasions. Each time Peter maintained that his "friends" had suggested that he help them by taking a few things out of the store. Peter did not seem to learn from his experience. His parents were able to keep the charges from becoming serious and were generally successful in isolating Peter from this group of "friends."

Peter's parents observed that he was skillful with his hands and liked crafts. They introduced him to the art of woodworking. Peter liked this work and the family helped him open a business making and selling his crafts. The family has found that it requires nearly continual supervision to keep Peter in the shop during business hours and to supervise all business transactions. He also needs to be gently guided in the evenings to prevent wayward activities. It requires the time of both parents as well as an aunt and uncle to supervise Peter's day.

Peter is proud of his business and perceives himself to be an independent adult. He enjoys his family and his contacts through his business. He would like a girl friend but does not seem overly troubled by his current inability to develop such a relationship.

When Peter came to the clinic he was readily diagnosed as having fetal alcohol syndrome based on his short stature, facial appearance, abnormal neurologic examination, and psychometric profile. The diagnosis had never been previously suggested to the parents, although they had worried about this possibility for many years.

Peter is seriously disabled although he did not qualify for any type of public assistance prior to his diagnosis with FAS and has had little understanding in his community. In spite of this, his family's enormous vigilance, energy and caring have prevented him from getting into any serious trouble and have provided him with a strong self image and pride in his abilities. Unfortunately, the energy required to manage Peter has taken its toll on his parents, who are reaching retirement age and are fearful that they will not be able to watch Peter as closely as needed in the future. His parents have not been able to find a halfway house for him.

MARY

Mary is a 43-year-old woman who has lived most her life in a variety of small to medium-sized communities. Both of her parents drank heavily on weekends and frequently on week nights, when alcohol was available. Her mother died before Mary was eight years old. Mary believed she died from cirrhosis of the liver or other alcohol-related internal problems. After the death of her mother, Mary was raised by several foster families, including an uncle and aunt.

Mary dropped out of school in the eighth grade and returned later to finish only the ninth grade. She had been held back one year, in the fifth grade, and it seemed that some of her promotions were due solely to the fact that she was in a special education track. She was in the ninth grade and not doing well when she had her first child at age 18.

Mary has given birth to four children, two boys and two girls. She had a miscarriage at age 27. Mary had two unstable marriages and vacillated in her drinking from heavy bingeing on weekends to regular drinking every night. Both of her husbands and her friends condoned and even encouraged heavy drinking on weekends. Whenever possible, though, she would drink heavily with friends on the weekends, usually in bars or at parties. She had participated in inpatient alcohol treatment programs twice, once in her mid-thirties and again at age 42. At the time of the interview, she had been abstinent for more than nine months. She had had some experience with Alcoholics Anonymous groups, but generally the lack of interest of her male partner was an impediment to staying in these groups. Mary had had her first experience with drinking at age 15.

When asked about her life in general, Mary became very thoughtful and quizzical. Her speech was slow and the thoughts seemed laborious. She said, "I always knew that I was different." She went on to recall that "I never felt that I fit in, and many things which went on around me, confused me. There were many things that I didn't understand in school, and school had very little purpose for me." When told of her diagnosis of possible FAS at age 43, Mary stated that she found the diagnosis "interesting." She said that "maybe that is why I do some of the things that I do." One of the things that she highlighted in her discussion was that she felt that she was a weak person. She felt that she was never able to follow through on her wishes and desires the way other people do.

At the time of the interview, her third husband was a recovering alcoholic. They had met in alcohol inpatient treatment. She worked as a domestic and he as a janitor for the alcohol treatment program. The two of them are supporting one another in their new life-style.

At age 43, Mary does not have custody of any of her four children. The oldest child, a girl, is married, has two children, and from all indications is living a normal life in a town several hundred miles away. The two middle children, both boys, are teenagers who have had various problems with school, both having been raised to a great extent in foster homes and in boarding schools for children with unstable family backgrounds. Only the younger of the two boys has needed special education, because he shows some signs of learning disabilities. The youngest child has been in foster placement for most of her life. She has been back and forth between Mary and foster homes four different times. Mary has a major goal of seeing three of her four children periodically and wants desperately to regain custody of her youngest child. Her hopes for the future are to remain sober, to be a good wife to her new husband, to get custody of the youngest child, and to watch her older children and her stepchildren grow.

BABY HERBERT'S MOTHER

Herbert was first seen on the second day of his life in the intensive care unit of a large children's hospital. He was born the day before at a community hospital and transferred because of his small size and intermittent bradycardia associated with a heart murmur.

Herbert was three weeks premature and small for his gestational age. He was in the 15th percentile for height and below the 3rd percentile for weight. His face was unusual. His eye slits (palpebral fissures) were very short. In addition, his upper lip was thin, his philtrum was thin, and his nose was short and upturned. He had a heart murmur compatible with a ventricular septal defect, and he had unusual creases on his palms suggesting unusual flexing of the hands in mid-gestation. His head circumference was small (3rd percentile), and his neurological exam was abnormal in that there was a poor suck and low tone.

The medical staff dysmorphologist determined that Herbert had fetal alcohol syndrome and called the referring physician with this information. The physician responded that the mother had been seen in an emergency room two weeks prior to delivery with acute gastritis and a high blood alcohol concentration. The physician said that she had had no previous suspicion that the mother had any problems with alcohol abuse. The mother was a 28-year-old accountant who had worked until shortly before delivery. Her husband was a mid-level manager in a technical field and had participated in his wife's prenatal care visits.

When the children's hospital staff (including physicians, nurses, and social worker) became aware of the FAS diagnosis, they were enraged with the mother, although they had not met her. They contacted child protective services and began to plan for the removal of the baby from his mother's care.

When Herbert's mother was released from the hospital herself and came to see her baby, she was appropriately concerned about the health of her child. She was soon overwhelmed by the hospital staff's hostile attitude and threatening approach. She responded to the accusations of fetal abuse by flatly denying any use or abuse of alcohol during her pregnancy. This led the hospital staff to view her as a liar and to see this as further proof that she was an unfit mother.

In fact, the hospital staff had no information at the time to indicate that Brenda (when sober) could not care for her child effectively, or that she had rationally understood that drinking during pregnancy could hurt her baby and yet continued to drink anyway. Denial of alcohol use and potential harm is common in those dependent on alcohol.

The hospital staff was helped to see that both the mother and the child were their patients. The recognition of FAS in the baby was an opportunity for positive intervention with his mother. This was a moment, if handled appropriately and supportively, when she might be ready to confront her alcohol dependence, thus improving her health, maximizing her ability to care for her child, and preventing fetal damage in future pregnancies.

REFERENCES

Dorris M. The Broken Cord. New York: Harper and Row, 1989.
Dorris M. Paper Trail: Essays. New York: HarperCollins, 1994.

4

Diagnosis and Clinical Evaluation of Fetal Alcohol Syndrome

Since the original description of fetal alcohol syndrome (FAS) approximately two decades ago, substantial progress has been made in developing specific criteria for delineating this syndrome. Nonetheless, a variety of key issues continue to sustain areas of controversy. The boundaries of the diagnosis, as well as the markers that should be used to delineate those boundaries, are perhaps the most vexing issues. Current discussions of FAS have also included discussions of a related condition known as "fetal alcohol effects." This latter condition has been variably defined, but often includes the concept that a subset of FAS features can occur and be related to a suspected maternal exposure to alcohol. Difficulties in obtaining an adequate history of alcohol intake, a widely recognized problem in medical evaluation, add to the complexity of this issue. The resolution of these issues is not trivial, for they have important implications for both patient care and social policy. Consequently, one charge of this committee was to evaluate existing diagnostic criteria and, in updating and expanding these, to consider the formulation of the best possible diagnostic guidelines, which could subsequently be used in epidemiologic, clinical, and basic research into this syndrome. In this context, it is helpful to step back and examine the process of diagnostic evaluation within its broadest context.

PURPOSE OF MEDICAL DIAGNOSES

A medical diagnosis serves several major purposes: to facilitate communication among clinicians; to facilitate communication between clinician and patient (including, in this instance, the parents of patients); to assist in the study of pathophysiology and etiology; and to guide treatment.

Providing a diagnostic label for a condition gives clinicians a common language that is useful in discussion. Diagnoses such as measles or fetal alcohol syndrome provide clinicians with a term that invokes a concept. On hearing this term, they can immediately call on an array of related facts and concepts that assist them in conveying information in a consistent manner. For the term to be useful to clinicians the diagnosis should be used in exactly the same way by everyone for several reasons: epidemiologic data can then be accurately collected, and patient records transferred from one site to another will contain information that can be interpreted accurately. Diagnoses are also used in order to conduct clinical research, with the long-term goal of understanding the mechanisms that cause a particular illness. For this purpose, it is equally important that diagnoses be consistent and accurate. Finally, diagnoses are used to assist clinicians in selecting appropriate treatments. Quite often, the process of differential diagnosis provides a road map that directs the clinician in the choice of treatment programs that otherwise may be quite different. In the differential diagnosis of acute abdominal pain, a diagnosis of appendicitis will send the patient to an operating room, whereas cystitis will lead to a prescription for medication.

USE OF DIAGNOSTIC CRITERIA

Because of the obvious importance of diagnosis in clinical medicine, during recent years nosologists have stressed the necessity of making the diagnostic process more objective and explicit. This improvement in the diagnostic process has often been implemented through the development of "diagnostic criteria." One of the earliest efforts in this direction was achieved by the American Heart Association, which developed criteria for defining the stages of cardiac failure. The most comprehensive effort produced to date was initiated by the Task Force on Nosology of the American Psychiatric Association, which completed a comprehensive revision in the third edition of its Diagnostic and Statistical Manual (known as DSM-III), published in 1980. In this manual, for the first time a comprehensive list of diagnoses for mental illness was defined through the use of explicit diagnostic criteria. This process led to a careful conceptualization of the best way to develop diagnostic criteria for specific illnesses.

STANDARDS FOR EVALUATING DIAGNOSTIC CRITERIA

Two requirements are typically used to evaluate diagnostic criteria. First, the criteria must be reliable. Second, they must be as valid as possible.

The concept of reliability refers to agreement among clinicians and consistency over time. In both cases, the essential feature is that the diagnosis be consistent and stable, so that good agreement occurs. Interrater reliability refers to the ability of two clinicians to look at the same phenomena and reach similar diagnostic conclusions. For example, two clinicians looking at a young patient with possible FAS would survey the clinical history, evaluate the facial features, examine any other ancillary data, and reach precisely the same diagnosis. Test-retest reliability refers to the ability to make the same diagnosis with time gaps between the assessment. Ideally, a child with FAS evaluated at 6 months, 12 months, 6 years, and 15 years of age would be given the same diagnosis even in the absence of information about previous clinicians' judgment.

Diagnostic criteria operationalize the steps that are used in making a diagnosis by delineating the particular features to be stressed. They are typically designed to be comprehensive and general, so that they can be applied at any point in the patient's history. The components that are used to make the diagnosis, such as the characteristic symptoms, are selected because good interrater agreement can be achieved for these specific symptoms. Once criteria are developed, their reliability can be assessed objectively through well-designed clinical studies that examine interrater or test-retest reliability. Statistical methods for measuring reliability have reached a mature state, and consensus has been reached by nosologists that reliability coefficients at a minimal level of 0.5 or 0.6 are acceptable, while coefficients of 0.7 through 0.9 are preferable.

Validity is the second important standard that is used to evaluate diagnostic criteria. Whereas reliability refers to precision of measurement or agreement, validity refers to the relevance or clinical utility of a set of diagnostic criteria. Theoretically, criteria can be highly reliable and yet totally invalid. If nosologists were to decide, for example, that height should be used as a criterion for diagnosing mental retardation, since it can be measured in a reliable manner, they would be choosing a criterion that had excellent reliability, but questionable validity. Clearly, therefore, it is important that diagnostic criteria contain components that are clinically meaningful and that lead to correct inferences about the nature of the pathological process.

Validity is usually divided into three components. Face validity means simply that the criteria selected conform to common sense; that is the criteria include features that are familiar to most clinicians and are based on some consensus that they are helpful. Construct validity refers to the fact that a diagnosis and its criteria conform to some conceptual construct or theory. For example, the construct of aberration in cell proliferation modulated by a variety of genetic, immunologic, toxic, and other mechanisms unifies the concept of cancer. One of the major issues for FAS diagnosis is the importance of documenting exposure to alcohol. Predictive validity is the third type of validity considered to be important. Predictive validity assists clinicians in making some prediction about the future. This prediction may involve decisions about treatment or guidance about prognosis.

ISSUES IN DECIDING ON DIAGNOSTIC CRITERIA

In addition to the well-documented guidelines of good reliability and validity, a number of practical considerations also inform decisions about diagnostic criteria. While reliability and validity set important standards that should be achieved in a good diagnostic system, the day-to-day process of deciding which specific signs and symptoms or other diagnostic indicators should be applied may depend on the clinical context in which a set of criteria is likely to be used. In the everyday world, diagnostic criteria are used for a variety of purposes.

A gatekeeping function is one practical purpose of diagnosis. That is, placing a patient in a diagnostic category confers both advantages and disadvantages. Sometimes these aspects work at cross-purposes to one another. For example, the diagnosis of FAS may validate a patient's disability and facilitate appropriate interventions and social benefits. On the other hand, the diagnosis may also be used to stigmatize and to create self-fulfilling prophecies about the future that could be detrimental to the patient and his or her family. Therefore, when diagnostic criteria are developed, nosologists must be sensitive to the various purposes for which these criteria will be used and choose the "gate" accordingly.

A descriptive function is a second important practical purpose of diagnostic criteria. Once criteria for an illness are defined, they are typically used to train appropriate clinicians to make that diagnosis. The increasing interest in making diagnoses more objective and reliable has led to the widespread use of diagnostic criteria in a variety of settings: by epidemiologists, third-party payers, forensic experts, and educators, as well as the clinicians for whom they were originally developed. The items selected for inclusion in the criteria are typically assumed by these various "consumers" to be the definitive description of the disorder. If signs or symptoms are not included in the criteria, they are often considered unimportant. In this context, therefore, the descriptive function is an addition to the gatekeeping function. For some illnesses, only one or two criteria may be needed to "enter the diagnostic gate," but more criteria would be needed to convey the clinical richness and complexity of a given disorder.

A final issue that arises in deciding on the explicit items to be used in diagnostic criteria is whether the conceptual construct should be narrow or broad. This issue is clearly related to both the gatekeeping function and the descriptive function. Decisions that are made within the context of this issue can have far-reaching implications. Setting criteria to a narrow window will improve the precision with which research on pathophysiology and etiology can be conducted by identifying rigorously defined groups. Such a strategy may be overly restrictive and result in research findings with poor generalizability to the population of individuals who may be suffering from the condition. On the other hand, if the window for diagnosis is set broadly reliability will be decreased, as will the precision of research, while generalizability is likely to be improved. There is no simple solution to the tension between these various goals, but the existence of this tension suggests the importance of attempting to identify a moderate position.

One solution to resolving the "narrow versus broad" issue is to create two sets of criteria, one to be used for research and the other for clinical applications. If this is done, then the research criteria are typically more narrow, while the clinical criteria are more broad.

SPECIFIC ISSUES TO BE ADDRESSED IN IDENTIFYING CRITERIA FOR FETAL ALCOHOL SYNDROME

In this context, a number of specific issues have been recognized as relevant in identifying appropriate criteria for fetal alcohol syndrome and related disorders. These issues have important implications for case definition, research, and treatment. They exist within the practical tensions described above, such as the gatekeeping function, the descriptive function, the virtue of narrow or broad definitions, and the use of criteria for research or clinical decisionmaking.

The key issues noted by the committee for identification of FAS include the following:

1. Should a documented history of exposure to alcohol be required for the diagnosis of FAS?
2. Which physical features should be used to define the disorder?
3. Can behavioral or cognitive features be used to define the disorder?
4. Is there a role for ancillary measures (e.g., magnetic resonance imaging [MRI]) in making the diagnosis?
5. Can criteria be designed to be used across the life span?
6. What is the relationship of so-called fetal alcohol effects to fetal alcohol syndrome?

Exposure to Alcohol

Although the criterion of exposure to alcohol appears easy to apply on the surface, it is in fact one of the most difficult issues in the study of fetal alcohol syndrome. It is well recognized that people are not always forthright about their history of alcohol intake, nor are they able to recall accurately the precise timing and severity of many different kinds of events from their past. A sensitive and specific biomarker of alcohol exposure could play an important role in this regard. This is discussed more fully in Chapter 7. The documentation of alcohol exposure in gestation is further complicated by the fact that some children who were exposed to alcohol during pregnancy were then subsequently adopted, so that the clinician cannot have direct access to the biological mother in order to obtain a history.

In addition, a clear consensus is not available concerning the amount of alcohol that can actually be toxic to the fetus or the relevance of standard definitions and diagnoses of alcohol abuse or dependence to the risk of having a child with FAS. Alcohol abuse is generally thought of either in terms of the social effects on an individual's life or, more rarely, in terms of the amount of intake. These two approaches to its definition do not always lead to mutually consistent conclusions. The requirement for documented indicators of physiological dependence provides a more objective definition, but may also be excessively narrow and stringent. Finally, the existing research literature appears to suggest that alcohol exerts its greatest toxic effect on central nervous system (CNS) development when given in large boluses. In human situations, this translates into drinking binges. Such binges may be more difficult to document historically and to time chronologically. The toxic effects of mild low-level alcohol intake are unclear and controversial. Chapter 2 contains a discussion of this in the animal literature and Chapter 7 will discuss the implications for prevention efforts. As Chapter 1 outlined, the committee focused its diagnostic criteria work in this chapter on the effects of exposure to large amounts of alcohol. Any conclusions made concerning the definition of alcohol exposure for FAS will have wide-reaching public health and social implications; hence, this a not a minor issue. The committee has considered the scientific literature and has a working definition of that level of exposure. This definition is flexible to accommodate new research findings.

Defining Physical Features

Historically FAS has been defined by growth deficiency, a pattern of facial anomalies, and indicators of brain dysfunction. Controversy swirls around how to measure each of these components and the weight to be given to each of them. Alcohol affects each of these factors along a spectrum from mild to severe injury, and further, each of these factors is affected by multiple environmental and genetic influences that are unrelated to alcohol exposure. For example, birth weight is related to gestational age, maternal nutritional state, and maternal size. Each of the craniofacial features can vary from distinctive to close to the normal range; overlap with other clinical syndromes, or reflect nonspecific family traits. To the extent that identification of these anomalies requires special expertise, the criteria will be less broadly useful in diagnostic settings that lack such expertise. Finally, evidence of brain maldevelopment as reflected, for example, by small cranial size also ranges from clear-cut changes to those within the normal range, and reflects both genetic and environmental influences. Cutoff points will inevitably be arbitrary, and population norms may vary over time and geographic location.

Behavioral or Cognitive Features

A variety of behavioral and cognitive features have been proposed as indicators of brain dysfunction in FAS. Examples include poor performance on tests of intelligence and educational achievement, impaired language development, poor impulse control, and problems with memory and judgment. At present, however, no consensus has been achieved as to which features are most appropriate for the diagnosis of FAS, or indeed whether any are appropriate. To some extent, these features mirror the problems noted for physical features. They too are on a continuum that ranges from normality to impaired, and they are also influenced by other antecedents such as parental intelligence, educational experience, impoverished postnatal environment, and other social and cultural influences. In addition, these cognitive and behavioral features are less specific to FAS than are the physical features; they tend to change with time, and they also tend to occur in association with a wide range of childhood neurodevelopmental and psychiatric conditions, for example, fragile X syndrome and attention-deficit hyperactivity disorder. Further, the teratogenic effects of alcohol on such cognitive and behavioral features are less well established through studies using rigorous experimental designs, although ample anecdotal evidence has been presented in the clinical literature.

Role of Ancillary Measures

Other indicators of the effects of alcohol on the brain may be provided through neuroimaging techniques such as computed tomography (CT) or magnetic resonance imaging (MRI). For example, recent studies suggest that well-documented cases of FAS may show a variety of abnormalities, such as callosal dysgenesis or agenesis or cerebellar hypoplasia. Further, MRI and CT can also provide a precise quantitative measure of brain volume, permitting more accurate and clinically meaningful assessment of microcephaly. Nonetheless, this technology is young; and consequently, normative data and the current evidentiary base are necessarily small. Consequently, the role of such ancillary measures is also controversial, and their utility in making a diagnosis of FAS is yet to be established.

Norms for human fetal growth, including fetal size, biparietal diameter, and placental growth, are being established based on serial examination of normal pregnancies using noninvasive ultrasound and three-dimensional imaging. Application of such normative standards to pregnancies at risk for FAS can be expected to increase our ability to recognize fetal growth retardation and may contribute to earlier recognition of FAS.

When the healthy human fetal growth curve is determined by serial ultrasound examinations of babies of normal size who go on to deliver at term, the fetal weight at each gestational age is greater than that described from birth weight data of babies delivering prematurely. Such new standards for intrauterine growth should increase the likelihood of recognizing intrauterine growth retardation earlier in pregnancy. In addition, it is possible that the introduction of three-dimensional imaging of placental volume will allow recognition of pregnancies that will develop fetal growth retardation several weeks earlier than such problems can now be diagnosed, by demonstrating reduced placental growth prior to recognizable fetal growth retardation (Wolf et al., 1989).

Diagnosis Across the Life Span

The indicators used to diagnose FAS were first codified in neonates, infants, and young children, but were then found to vary across the life span. The recognition that phenotype varies with age makes it more difficult to identify appropriate features for inclusion in diagnostic criteria that are not age specific. For example, some craniofacial anomalies may be less evident at birth, become more conspicuous during early infancy and childhood, and often diminish or even disappear during adolescence and adulthood. Furthermore, the decreased cranial size and reduced birth weight originally considered to be hallmarks of FAS have become less pathognomonic in the view of some clinicians who see children with FAS. As is always the case in defining growth disturbance, this may not be a striking feature, and there will always be cases that fall within normal ranges. Therefore, identification of these anomalies will be easier or more difficult depending on the age at which the child is assessed.

Relationship of Fetal Alcohol Effects to Fetal Alcohol Syndrome

The term fetal alcohol effects, as described below, was originally developed to describe abnormalities observed in animal studies, but was quickly adopted by clinicians. It soon came to be widely used to refer to behavioral and cognitive problems occurring in children exposed to alcohol in utero without the typical diagnostic features. Because of the difficulties inherent in measuring exposure to alcohol, coupled with the difficulties inherent in quantifying or demarcating behavioral and cognitive problems, the precision of this terminology (never very exact) has gradually been reduced. Many believe that the term should be abandoned altogether (Aase et al., 1995, Sokol and Clarren, 1989), although the term is still widely used.

EVOLUTION OF THE DIAGNOSIS OF
FETAL ALCOHOL SYNDROME

The clinical recognition of virtually every multiple malformation syndrome has begun with a case report describing a small number of individuals. The patients in such a report typically have a highly similar (but not identical) set of anomalies that is made unique from previously described syndromes by the inclusion of some very rare anomalies or by an unusual association of more common anomalies. Such a new syndrome then evolves as more patients are recognized. Although the hallmark features of a new disorder generally do not change over time, the list of associated features is usually modified and revised by further clinical experience.

When the etiology of a syndrome can be measured independently of clinical presentation (i.e., through chromosomal studies, metabolic testing, or pathologic findings), its presentation generally expands to include patients who do not have the "classic" physical characteristics of syndromic expression. Additionally, some patients who had appeared to have the syndrome on clinical grounds will be excluded from the condition because the independent measure of the disorder is negative (phenocopies). In multiple malformation syndromes due to teratogens, phenotypic variability would be even more likely than in genetic disorders since variable patterns of dose exposure and frequency of exposure, combined with variations in fetal and maternal metabolism, should produce varying clinical presentations. Clinical geneticists and dysmorphologists have been reluctant to establish rigid case definitions for any birth defect syndrome. Rightly or wrongly, there has always been concern that imposing rigid diagnostic criteria on a syndrome with assumed phenotypic variability would tie clinicians' hands and prevent further description of the syndrome's full presentation.

Fetal alcohol syndrome does not represent the full spectrum of alcohol teratogenesis, but rather comprises a subset of patients who were exposed to alcohol and who have a unique recognizable pattern of malformation. The condition has evolved from initial case reports by Lemoine in 1968 and Jones and Smith in 1973. The hallmark features of the disorder were a characteristic set of facial features, evidence of growth deficiency, evidence of structural or organic brain dysfunction, and occasionally, associated malformations of organ systems, such as the heart or skeleton. Of these anomalies, the facial gestalt was the most clinically unique, while CNS dysfunction was the most significant.

Over the last 25 years, clinical observations from a dozen countries with thousands of patients have confirmed that alcohol exposure in utero can produce fetal alcohol syndrome as defined. However, the way each aspect of the phenotype is defined and assessed has been refined in terms both of descriptors per se and of presentation over a patient's life span.

The progress in refining the FAS diagnosis can be traced by reviewing Clarren and Smith (1978), who summarized the available clinical reports from 1973 to 1976, and the reports from the fetal alcohol workshops of the Research Society on Alcoholism in 1980 and 1989 (Rosett, 1980; Sokol and Clarren, 1989).

Experience with the FAS diagnosis remains somewhat circular at this time which is a typical problem in clinical syndromology and hardly unique to FAS. Clinical experts assert that certain patients have fetal alcohol syndrome and the abnormalities found in those patients are then used to refine the diagnosis. A truer case definition will be established only when a reliable biologic marker for alcohol teratogenesis is found or when a diagnostic tool is developed that can demonstrate high sensitivity and specificity in identifying dysmorphic individuals who were exposed in utero to potentially teratogenic doses of alcohol.

At present, the facial anomalies observed in FAS remain the most unique feature of the disorder (see Figure 1 in Chapter 1). No one can receive an FAS diagnosis without an experienced clinician's assertion that the face, *when taken as a whole*, appears to be the FAS face. Unfortunately, the full complement of anomalies that produce this facial appearance has been difficult to reduce to verbal descriptors, and a reliable listing of properly weighted and verbally defined abnormalities has not yet been fully developed. Several Centers for Disease Control (CDC)-sponsored FAS projects are working to develop screening check lists. Photographic pattern recognition has proven up to now to be a better way to teach the facial gestalt of FAS. Generally, the anomalies that seem to create the FAS appearance are localized to the central facial region and form a sort of "T." The upper horizontal bar of the T is formed by the eyes and inner canthal region. In this area, the palpebral fissures (eye slits) are short, usually measuring well below -2 SD (standard deviation) for age, while the inner canthal distance is more variable and generally is normal for age or reflective of general family appearance unrelated to an alcohol effect. (It should be noted that population standards for palpebral fissures can be different in some ethnic groups; this can cause difficulties in making the diagnosis if this is not recognized.) Ptosis, high lateral arched eyebrows, and epicanthal folds are associated anomalies that may be present but do not define the horizontal bar without the shortened palpebral fissures. The vertical bar of the T is defined by the nose and philtral (premaxillary) region. In this area, the philtral furrows are flattened or hypoplastic, and the upper lip (the vermilion) is thinned. The medial midface, the maxillary area abutting the nose, is also flattened. At this time, no standards have been established for when features are specifically short enough, small enough, or flat enough for a true case definition. Yet all of these features seem necessary for the FAS facial gestalt to be present. Other anomalies of the mandible and outer ears may be seen, but do not seem to contribute to or detract from the FAS facial gestalt.

No single expression of structural or functional brain damage is universal or pathognomonic when patients with the FAS face and a clear history of substantial alcohol exposure are reviewed. Evidence of abnormality in this field may be structural, neurologic, or functional. Microcephaly was emphasized as a necessary marker for structural damage in early reports, but many, if not most, clinicians who diagnose a lot of children with FAS do not regard this as a necessary finding now. Only 16 autopsies of humans with FAS have been published; these suggest a diversity of lesions in multiple sites (West and Pierce, 1986). CT and MRI images of the brain in FAS patients have been reported to display mild changes in ventricular size, disruptions in structure such as hypoplasia or agenesis of the corpus callosum, and decreased cerebellar size. Neurologic evidence for brain damage may include seizures, abnormalities in muscle tone, tremors, abnormalities in coordination, neurosensory hearing loss, or visual anomalies stemming from small optic globes.

FAS finally can be characterized by behavioral or cognitive problems that are thought to result from organic brain damage, are not easily related to genetic background or environmental influences, and are resistant to improvement with traditionally effective intervention techniques. In most patients, neurodevelopmental problems are complex and multifaceted; they include cognitive delays (but not necessarily into the mental deficiency range); attention problems that do not seem to be classical attention-deficit hyperactivity disorder; learning disability, with better strength in reading and language, and poorer ability in math; and speech and language delays that are most apparent in the use of complex speech idiom and poor understanding of the meaning of paragraphs. There are frequently problems with reasoning and judgment often recognized as failure to learn from experience or to develop a logical approach to tasks of any type (e.g., social, moral, or academic).

The initial cases of fetal alcohol syndrome were often culled from early assessments of children failing to thrive. Growth deficiency has historically been regarded as a major feature of the disorder. Abundant research in humans and in animals demonstrates that alcohol can have adverse impact on length and weight both prenatally and postnatally. However, it is probable that the major impact on fetal growth comes from alcohol exposure in the last half of gestation, whereas the facial anomalies and brain problems associated with alcohol teratogenesis are more likely of earlier gestational origin. However, many reports have noted that patients may present with the face of FAS and evidence of brain dysfunction of prenatal origin but have growth that is within the normal range. Some of these patients were born with height, weight, or head circumference within normal ranges. Others were well below normal ranges at birth but "caught up" in adolescence; this has been noted particularly with regard to weight in females. Should the FAS definition be adjusted for such patients? This issue is not resolved as yet.

LONGITUDINAL PERSPECTIVES ON THE FAS DIAGNOSIS

In general, experts have little difficulty making an FAS diagnosis in children between the ages of 2 and 11 years. Prior to age 2, some children with FAS do not show all the facial features in the vertical bar of the T or do not have clear evidence of CNS dysfunction of prenatal origin.

After puberty, catch-up growth is common, and children who had been light for weight and below -2 SD for height and weight accelerate into the more normal range. Often the vertical bar of the T disappears again. Historical growth data and prepubertal photographs are often needed to establish an FAS diagnosis in these older patients.

The fact that this syndrome is most easily diagnosed in a specific period of life is not unique to FAS. Many syndromes become easier or more difficult to diagnose with increasing patient age. For example, the Wiedemann-Beckwith syndrome is defined by macrosomia at birth and large viscera. Typically the tongue is quite large and there is an omphalocele present in the newborn period. In infants this is a readily apparent disorder, but as the child ages organ size and overall height normalize. After puberty the syndrome is extremely subtle and would generally not be considered without the neonatal description. The Prader-Willi syndrome is defined by hypotonia in infancy, mental retardation, hypogonadism, and progressive obesity in childhood. While the hyoptonia, hypogonadism and the minor anomalies are present in infancy, the diagnosis (prior to the recent advent of chromosomal testing) was withheld until the obesity and developmental delay become apparent in the second or third year of life. Similarly, the hallmark of Fragile-X syndrome is testicular enlargement which is generally not found until after puberty. Prior to the discovery of the genetic marker, Fragile-X syndrome was rarely diagnosed until the second decade of life.

DIAGNOSTIC CATEGORIES

One of the key charges to the committee was to review and evaluate the diagnostic criteria for FAS and related conditions. The committee studied the previous diagnostic criteria and felt that some of the issues confusing the clinical and research communities could be resolved with fairly minor changes in the diagnostic categories and criteria. These new criteria can be found in Table 4-1.

The diagnostic criteria for FAS as described in the preceding section are found under Category 1, FAS with confirmed maternal alcohol exposure. A diagnosis is placed in this category when appropriate anomalies are found in face, brain, *and* growth, *and* a clear history of alcohol exposure is obtained. The committee currently defines the relevant history as one of a pattern of excessive intake characterized by substantial, regular intake or heavy episodic drinking. Evidence of this pattern may include: frequent episodes of intoxication, development of tolerance or withdrawal, social problems related to drinking, legal problems related to drinking, engaging in physically hazardous behavior while drinking, or alcohol-related medical problems such as hepatic disease. It is anticipated that patients in this category would remain the template for further delineation of the condition.

Category 2, FAS without confirmed maternal alcohol exposure, is assigned to patients with all the clear phenotypic features necessary for an FAS diagnosis but without a confirmed history of alcohol exposure. Many patients with FAS are in foster or adoptive placements and their prenatal exposure histories are unavailable. In other cases, the birth mother honestly cannot recall the specifics of her alcohol use in gestation or remains in denial of her alcohol abuse. It is unfair to deny these patients the clinical benefits of a medical diagnosis, but it also seems imprudent to combine their cases with those in the first category, FAS with confirmed maternal alcohol exposure, when carrying out some forms of research. Therefore, it is recommended that they be grouped separately.

It also remains theoretically possible that individuals might be found with the full FAS phenotype and a confirmed negative history of gestational alcohol exposure. (Phenocopies do exist for nearly every condition.) Although we are not aware that this situation has arisen yet, such cases should not be considered in category 2. They do not have FAS.

Category 3, partial FAS with confirmed maternal alcohol exposure, is assigned to patients with a confirmed exposure to substantial amounts of alcohol in gestation, some components of the facial features of FAS, and any of the following: evidence of growth deficiency, CNS neurodevelopmental abnormalities, or a complex pattern of behavioral and cognitive abnormalities. This diagnostic category allows an FAS diagnosis to be given to someone who would not receive a Category 1 diagnosis, FAS with confirmed maternal alcohol exposure. This diagnosis could be particularly useful, for example, for some patients who present for diagnosis as an adult. The natural history of FAS is such that some of the "hallmark" indicators used in infancy or childhood are not maintained into adolescence or adulthood. For example, facial dysmorphia can become less distinct and some adolescents, particularly females, gain weight into or above normal ranges. Absent good medical records of growth retardation at birth and early infancy, an FAS diagnosis otherwise could not be given without Category 3. This diagnosis could also be given to those young children whose growth metrics are within normal ranges, which some studies suggest can occur if the mother cuts down her alcohol exposure in the third trimester. This diagnosis can also be used as a "holding" category as a means to defer a diagnosis of Category 1, FAS with confirmed maternal history of alcohol exposure, until more data collection or evaluation, including documentation as to whether behavioral and cognitive abnormalities persist over time, can support a more definitive diagnosis. In the newborn, for example, there is some controversy whether some behavioral abnormalities, such as abnormalities of state regulation, indicate or predict long-term dysfunction due to fetal alcohol exposure. In such cases, documentation of abnormalities over time would be important.

The naming of this diagnostic category was challenging for the committee, who found no perfect solution. Terms considered were probable, partial, and atypical. "Probable" was unsatisfactory, because it denotes uncertainty about the etiology of the condition and because of concerns that appropriate services or reimbursement for these services would not be made for a "probable" condition. The committee intends for this diagnostic category to include people with signs and symptoms attributable to significant prenatal alcohol exposure and who need medical, social services, and other attention. "Atypical" has recently been dis-

TABLE 4-1   Diagnostic Criteria for Fetal Alcohol Syndrome (FAS) and
Alcohol-Related Effects

Fetal Alcohol Syndrome
1. FAS with confirmed maternal alcohol exposure[a]
A. Confirmed maternal alcohol exposure[a]
B. Evidence of a characteristic pattern of facial anomalies that includes features such as short palpebral fissures and abnormalities in the premaxillary zone (e.g., flat upper lip, flattened philtrum, and flat midface)
C. Evidence of growth retardation, as in at least one of the following:
   — low birth weight for gestational age
   — decelerating weight over time not due to nutrition
   — disproportional low weight to height
D. Evidence of CNS neurodevelopmental abnormalities, as in at least one of the following:
   — decreased cranial size at birth
   — structural brain abnormalities (e.g., microcephaly, partial or complete agenesis of the corpus callosum, cerebellar hypoplasia)
   — neurological hard or soft signs (as age appropriate), such as impaired fine motor skills, neurosensory hearing loss, poor tandem gait, poor eye-hand coordination

2. FAS without confirmed maternal alcohol exposure
B, C, and D as above

3. Partial FAS with confirmed maternal alcohol exposure
A. Confirmed maternal alcohol exposure[a]
B. Evidence of some components of the pattern of characteristic facial anomalies

Either C or D or E

C. Evidence of growth retardation, as in at least one of the following:
   — low birth weight for gestational age
   — decelerating weight over time not due to nutrition
   — disproportional low weight to height
D. Evidence of CNS neurodevelopmental abnormalities, as in:
   — decreased cranial size at birth
   — structural brain abnormalities (e.g., microcephaly, partial or complete agenesis of the corpus callosum, cerebellar hypoplasia)
   — neurological hard or soft signs (as age appropriate) such as impaired fine motor skills, neurosensory hearing loss, poor tandem gait, poor eye-hand coordination
E. Evidence of a complex pattern of behavior or cognitive abnormalities that are inconsistent with developmental level and cannot be explained by familial background or environment alone, such as learning difficulties; deficits in school performance; poor impulse control; problems in social perception; deficits in higher level receptive and expressive language; poor capacity for abstraction or metacognition; specific deficits in mathematical skills; or problems in memory, attention, or judgment

Alcohol-Related Effects
Clinical conditions in which there is a history of maternal alcohol exposure,[a,b] and where clinical or animal research has linked maternal alcohol ingestion to an observed outcome.

There are two categories, which may co-occur. If both diagnoses are present, then both diagnoses should be rendered:

4. Alcohol-related birth defects (ARBD)
List of congenital anomalies, including malformations and dysplasias

Cardiac	Atrial septal defects	Aberrant great vessels
	Ventricular septal defects	Tetralogy of Fallot
Skeletal	Hypoplastic nails	Clinodactyly
	Shortened fifth digits	Pectus excavatum and carinatum
	Radioulnar synostosis	Klippel-Feil syndrome
	Flexion contractures	Hemivertebrae
	Camptodactyly	Scoliosis
Renal	Aplastic, dysplastic,	Ureteral duplications
	hypoplastic kidneys	Hydronephrosis
	Horseshoe kidneys	
Ocular	Strabismus	Refractive problems secondary to small globes
	Retinal vascular anomalies	
Auditory	Conductive hearing loss	Neurosensory hearing loss
Other	Virtually every malformation has been described in some patient with FAS. The etiologic specificity of most of these anomalies to alcohol teratogenesis remains uncertain.	

5. Alcohol-related neurodevelopmental disorder (ARND)
Presence of:

A. Evidence of CNS neurodevelopmental abnormalities, as in any one of the following:
— decreased cranial size at birth
— structural brain abnormalities (e.g., microcephaly, partial or complete agenesis of the corpus callosum, cerebellar hypoplasia)
— neurological hard or soft signs (as age appropriate), such as impaired fine motor skills, neurosensory hearing loss, poor tandem gait, poor eye-hand coordination

and/or:

B. Evidence of a complex pattern of behavior or cognitive abnormalities that are inconsistent with developmental level and cannot be explained by familial background or environment alone, such as learning difficulties; deficits in school performance; poor impulse control; problems in social perception; deficits in higher level receptive and expressive language; poor capacity for abstraction or metacognition; specific deficits in mathematical skills; or problems in memory, attention, or judgment

---

[a]A pattern of excessive intake characterized by substantial, regular intake or heavy episodic drinking. Evidence of this pattern may include frequent episodes of intoxication, development of tolerance or withdrawal, social problems related to drinking, legal problems related to drinking, engaging in physically hazardous behavior while drinking, or alcohol-related medical problems such as hepatic disease.

[b]As further research is completed and as, or if, lower quantities or variable patterns of alcohol use are associated with ARBD or ARND, these patterns of alcohol use should be incorporated into the diagnostic criteria.

carded by DSM-IV and the committee did not think that these patients were "not typical." In fact, all of their signs and symptoms are typical of FAS. "Partial" denotes, to some people, that the condition might not be as severe, which the committee did not wish to imply. The committee settled on the use of "partial" despite these reservations. This category, and its name, should remain flexible. As further research reveals the range of the manifestations of FAS, this diagnosis should evolve to be consonant with new data. This diagnosis can be used to categorize such patients for future use in studying and understanding the condition.

The term fetal alcohol effects (FAE) was initially proposed (Clarren and Smith, 1978) as a term for use when an adverse birth outcome could be proven to be related to alcohol exposure in utero. Generally, this term is properly used in animal models of alcohol teratogenesis and in large prospective group studies of humans exposed to alcohol prenatally. The term was not meant for use with individual patients. Terms such as "suspected fetal alcohol effect" and "possible fetal alcohol effect" were suggested as entries on differential diagnostic lists, but this approach has not been well understood. Later, the term alcohol-related birth defects was suggested for clinical use with this category of patient (Sokol and Clarren, 1989). This term presents clinical problems because most patients who seek diagnosis and do not have FAS, but were alcohol-exposed, do not have major malformations of organs; rather, they have evidence of CNS neurodevelopmental abnormality. The term "birth defects" generally is understood by most lay people to refer to gross structural anomalies, although the March of Dimes defines birth defects as abnormalities of either structure or function.

The committee believes that it may be helpful to subdivide this patient group of possible prenatal *alcohol-related effects* into two groups listed in Table 4-1 as categories 4 and 5. Category 4, "alcohol-related birth defects" (ARBD), is reserved for patients with physical anomalies, and category 5, "alcohol-related neurodevelopmental disorder" (ARND), is reserved for patients with neurodevelopmental problems. These diagnostic categories include clinical conditions for which clinical or animal research has linked maternal alcohol ingestion to an observed outcome. A history of confirmed maternal alcohol exposure is required for these diagnoses. The relevant history remains as defined for FAS, but the committee notes that as further research is completed and as, or if, lower quantities or variable patterns of alcohol use are associated with ARBD or ARND, these patterns of alcohol use should be incorporated into the diagnostic criteria. These final two diagnostic categories are intended to convey some degree of uncertainty whether prenatal alcohol exposure caused the adverse effects documented in an individual patient, or whether other factors were causative in this case. Whereas patients in categories 1, 2 and, 3 are mutually exclusive, patients could be in both categories 4 and 5. Because of the variability in the specific presentation of FAS, ARBD, or ARND, these diagnoses are most valuable clinically if accompanied by a description of the specific problems experienced at the time by the patient. Only with such data will FAS, ARBD, and ARND be better understood.

DIFFERENTIAL DIAGNOSIS

While the "classic" presentation of fetal alcohol syndrome is distinct and can be readily distinguished from other disorders by an expert, even an expert may have difficulty confirming the diagnosis of FAS when the phenotype is "incomplete" or "atypical." Syndromes that have been confused with fetal alcohol syndrome are conditions that feature growth deficiencies and facial anomalies that are suggestive of, but different overall from, FAS. Examples of conditions confused with FAS because of somewhat similar appearance are Aarskog syndrome, Williams syndrome, Noonan's syndrome, Dubowitz syndrome, Bloom syndrome, fetal hydantoin syndrome, maternal PKU (phenylketonuria) fetal effects, and fetal toluene syndrome.

Other syndromes are confused with FAS because of similarities in complex cognitive and behavioral profiles, although the external phenotype is not really similar to FAS. Examples of conditions confused with FAS because of somewhat similar behavioral profiles are fragile X syndrome, velocardiofacial syndrome, Turner's syndrome, and Opitz syndrome.

CLINICAL UTILITY OF FAS, ARBD, AND ARND DIAGNOSES

In addition to the gatekeeping functions described for any diagnosis, identifying children with FAS or possible alcohol-related effects provides additional benefits to the mother, the child, and society. These are elaborated in Chapters 7 and 8 but can be summarized here. A comment about who should make this diagnosis needs to be made first, however. The committee believes that FAS, ARBD, and ARND will continue to be difficult diagnoses in many cases. The committee believes that a trained clinician can make the diagnosis for purposes of screening and referral but that a medical diagnosis of FAS remains the purview of dysmorphologists and clinical geneticists.

Prevention

The early identification of a child with FAS can be theoretically used as a marker that will lead to interventions with the mother for her own treatment and for the prevention of births of subsequent children with FAS. The diagnosis of FAS should stimulate efforts to lead the mother into sobriety. This is the best chance to prevent alcohol-related trauma and disease in the mother, increase the chance that she will be able to mother her child, decrease foster placement, and prevent the birth of more children with FAS. Chapter 7 contains further discussion of this issue.

Prevention of Secondary Disabilities

Children with FAS or ARND have impairments that cannot be normalized but possibly can be improved with appropriate interventions, and they can possibly be made worse when ignored or misunderstood. Generally, the diagnosis of FAS or ARND helps parents, educators, and others to understand that the child "can't" perform as opposed to "won't" perform. This change in awareness can prevent misinterpretation of the child's behavior and avoid inappropriate discipline and punishment. The diagnosis can lead to treatment plans that center around and support the child and prevent him or her from getting into situations that could lead to inappropriate behavior. Although cognitive problems are unavoidable, depression, anxiety, anger, antisocial behavior, and isolation do not need to result from this disorder.

Recognizing the syndrome and diagnosing it correctly can be helpful to individuals at any age. There have been no studies to demonstrate that secondary disabilities are better prevented if the diagnosis is made in the birth to three-year versus four- to seven-year period, but most professionals believe that the diagnosis becomes increasingly less effective in maximizing outcomes if the disorder is left unrecognized into adolescence.

RECOMMENDATIONS: DIAGNOSTIC CRITERIA

The committee-revised diagnostic criteria aim to increase clarity, rigor, and consistency by expanding the traditional designations of fetal alcohol syndrome and other possible alcohol-related effects. The key recommendations inherent in this new diagnostic scheme include the following:

• preserving the criteria for FAS diagnosis but now specifying whether or not prenatal alcohol exposure is documented;
• subdividing the diagnosis of other alcohol-related effects to distinguish physical anomalies from neurobehavioral and cognitive deficits, which can occur separately; and
• adoption and use of the revised criteria for classification and diagnosis by clinical and research professionals in the field.

Research recommendations include

• research to evaluate the utility, reliability, and validity of this scheme for classification and diagnosis;
• research, both cross-sectional and longitudinal, to assess the characteristics and clinical expression of these syndromes across the life span, particularly after adolescence;

- investigation of the differences in expression and specificity of behavioral and cognitive deficits in FAS and ARND;
- research to identify potential structural or functional brain abnormalities and other neurobiological indices that may be associated with, or distinguish, FAS, ARBD, or ARND, and to relate these abnormalities and indices to cognitive and behavioral correlates;
- further clinical research, as well as research using animal models, to examine the adverse developmental effects of prenatal alcohol exposure, and to develop more specific biologic markers for diagnosis (e.g., biomarkers to confirm maternal alcohol exposure, endocrine signals, imaging techniques); and
- consideration of the potential role of fetal alcohol exposure, as appropriate, in developmental disability studies in general.

REFERENCES

Aase JM, Jones KL, Clarren SK. Do We Need the Term "FAE"? Pediatrics 1995; 95:428-430.

American Psychiatric Association. Diagnostic and Statistical Manual of Mental Disorders: 3rd Edition. Washington, DC. 1980.

Clarren SK, Smith DW. The fetal alcohol syndrome. New England Journal of Medicine 1978; 298:1063-1067.

Jones KL, Smith DW. Recognition of the fetal alcohol syndrome in early infancy. Lancet 1973; 2:999-1001.

Lemoine P, Harouseau H, Borteryu JT, Menuet JC. Les enfants des parents alcooliques: Anomalies observees apropos de 127 cas. Ouest Medical 1968; 21:476-482.

Rosett HL. A clinical perspective of the Fetal Alcohol Syndrome. Alcoholism: Clinical and Experimental Research 1980; 4:119-122.

Sokol RJ, Clarren SK. Guidelines for use of terminology describing the impact of prenatal alcohol on the offspring. Alcoholism: Clinical and Experimental Research 1989; 13:597-598.

West JR, Pierce DR. Perinatal alcohol exposure and neuronal damage. Alcohol and Brain Development. J.R. West, (ed.). New York: Oxford University Press, 1986.

Wolf H, Oosting H, Treffers PE. Second-trimester placental volume measurement by ultrasound: Prediction of fetal outcome. American Journal of Obstetrics and Gynecology 1989; 160:121-126.

5

Epidemiology and Surveillance of Fetal Alcohol Syndrome

The success of any public health program can be measured by comparing the incidence or prevalence of a particular societal problem before that program was implemented with its incidence or prevalence after implementation. Such data are also important for estimating the societal impact of these disorders and are crucial at the initial stages of planning, organizing, and implementing prevention programs aimed at the general population as well as at specific at-risk populations (Beauchamp, 1980). The previous chapter discusses criteria for diagnosing FAS, ARBD, and ARND. That chapter points out that diagnostic criteria serve many purposes. So, too, do epidemiology and surveillance. In addition to the important reasons outlined above, it is important to survey FAS so that children identified can receive appropriate medical care, social services, and educational interventions. Epidemiology and surveillance of fetal alcohol syndrome (FAS), alcohol-related birth defects (ARBD), and alcohol-related neurodevelopmental disorder (ARND) are ongoing but are currently hampered by inconsistent methods and criteria for gathering the appropriate data. The chapter first describes estimates of the incidence and prevalence of FAS as reported in the published literature and as measured in three main ways. The chapter then discusses methodologic issues in FAS surveillance.

INCIDENCE AND PREVALENCE OF FAS, ARBD, ARND

The literature on the epidemiology of FAS and ARBD or ARND is extensive and complicated by differences in the definition of outcomes in this evolving field. Although prospectively gathered FAS incidence rates have been published in more than 20 different studies (see Abel and Sokol, 1987, 1991; Abel, in press), many of the estimates from the United States are based on high-risk populations living in lower-socioeconomic urban areas.

The incidence of FAS has been estimated from data of three main types: information collected passively for another or for many purposes, such as birth defects registries; information gathered either retrospectively or prospectively from hospital or clinic-based populations, including subjects in controlled epidemiologic studies of the effects of maternal substance abuse (which frequently measure the incidence or prevalence of traits or characteristics associated with FAS, not the incidence of FAS itself); and population-based active case ascertainment. A brief review of the literature of the incidence and prevalence of FAS and other possible alcohol-related effects follows. We have attempted to map findings to current terminology (see Chapter 4). Where this was not possible, we describe the diagnostic category employed but have avoided using fetal alcohol effects (FAE) or ARBD as they had been used historically (i.e., to designate other than FAS). The sections are organized according to the general methodological approach as specified above.

Registry-Based Studies

The Centers for Disease Control and Prevention monitors the rate of FAS in two birth defects surveillance programs. Chavez et al. (1988) reviewed the recording of major congenital malformations in CDC's Birth Defects Monitoring Program (BDMP). Cases were identified based on hospital discharge diagnoses using codes from the International Classification of Diseases, ninth edition (ICD-9-CM; U.S. Department of Health and Human Services, 1991a). Code 760.71 is "noxious influences affecting fetus via placenta or breast milk, specifically alcohol; includes fetal alcohol syndrome."

Data were collected in more than 1,500 hospitals across the United States from 1980 through 1986. The overall rate of FAS was 2.97 per 1,000 for Native Americans, 0.6 per 1,000 for African Americans, 0.09 for Caucasians, 0.08 for Hispanics, and 0.03 for Asians (Chavez et al., 1988). As might be expected, the rates of FAS ascertained from a birth certificate registry system were much lower than those for the clinic-based FAS-specific studies discussed later. The registry rate reported is about 1 per 10,000 rather than 1 to 2 per 1,000 as documented in epidemiologic studies.

A subsequent CDC article on data from the BDMP estimated the overall incidence of FAS from 1979 to 1993 at 0.22 per 1,000 (CDC, 1995a). For 1992 alone, however, the rate was 0.37 per 1,000 (CDC, 1993a), and for 1993 it was 0.67 per 1,000 (CDC, 1995a); these rates are substantially higher than in previous years. According to the CDC, this increase is leading to a study to examine the sensitivity and specificity of the monitoring system.

The CDC's Metropolitan Atlanta Congenital Defects Program (MACDP) is a population-based registry that identifies children diagnosed with birth defects during the neonatal and infancy periods. The program monitors all births in a five-county area in and around metropolitan Atlanta. In contrast to the BDMP, the MACDP uses multiple data sources, including hospital discharge data, medical records, and birth certificates. From 1989 through 1992, the MACDP identified an overall rate of FAS of 0.23 case per 1,000 (CDC, 1995b).

Other geographic regions, for example the states of California and Iowa, have birth defects registry systems. In general, the surveillance of FAS is similar in these other systems. Information on birth defects incidence and prevalence at the national level is inadequate and FAS is no exception. Birth registry systems that are used in the absence of active case identification or case-finding initiatives are not adequate approaches for producing estimates of FAS. Results are based on indicators at birth or, in the case of prevalence studies, only on indicators at a particular age. Given also that FAS is a complex diagnosis (see Chapter 4), it may go unrecognized at birth (Little et al., 1990). Thus, registry-based estimates of FAS prevalence can be expected to be gross underestimates.

Clinic-Based Studies

Studies that have produced rates, or estimated rates, of the incidence of FAS have been carried out in a number of countries (see Table 5-1). Many of these are based on populations seen in hospitals or clinics. These data can be collected prospectively or reviewed retrospectively. In Sweden the rate of FAS was found to be 1.7 per 1,000 births, and the rate of what seem to be ARBD and ARND 1.7 per 1,000, yielding an overall rate of 3.4 per 1,000 for diagnosable alcohol-related abnormalities (Olegard et al., 1979).

Early retrospective studies in France identified 2.9 FAS children per 1,000 births (Dehaene et al., 1977) and later 1.4 per 1,000 births (Dehaene et al., 1981). More recently, Dehaene and colleagues categorized FAS and possible alcohol-related effects severity into Types I, II, and III, with Type III being the most severe effects (i.e., FAS). In monitoring 13,118 births from 1986 to 1990, Type III FAS was estimated at 1.2 per 1,000 births. Types I and II (ARBD) were estimated at 4.8 per 1,000 births. This produced a combination ARBD rate of 6.0 per 1,000 in northern France (Dehaene et al., 1991).

Retrospectively gathered data invariably result in higher estimates (Abel and Sokol, 1987). For example, in contrast to these retrospective studies, prospective clinic-based studies in Australia, Canada, Finland, Switzerland, and the United Kingdom have failed to document any cases of FAS (Abel and Sokol, 1987, 1991).

In the United States, incidence rates vary widely depending on study site. Hanson et al. (1978) reported an incidence rate of 1.3 FAS children per 1,000 births for Seattle, Washington. This figure represented two African-American FAS babies born in a sample of 1,529 predominately Caucasian mothers. In the

TABLE 5-1 Prevalence of Fetal Alcohol Syndrome (FAS), Alcohol-Related Birth Defects (ARBD), and Alcohol-Related Neurodevelopmental Disorder (ARND), and Total in Selected Previous Studies

| Studies | | | Rate per 1,000 | | |
Type	Study	Locale	FAS	ARND/ARBD	[a]
Clinic based	Olgard et al. (1979)	Sweden	1.7	1.7	3.3
Clinic based	Dehaene et al. (1977)	France	2.9	—	—
Clinic based	Dehaene et al. (1981)	France	1.4	—	—
Clinic based	Dehaene et al. (1991)	France	1.2	—	6.0
Clinic based	Hanson et al. (1978)	U.S. (Seattle)	1.3	—	5.9
Clinic based	Hingson et al. (1977)	U.S. (Boston)	0.6	—	—
Clinic based	Ouellette et al. (1977)	U.S. (Boston)	3.1	—	—
Clinic based	Sokol et al. (1980)	U.S. (Cleveland)	0.6	—	—
Clinic based	Sokol et al. (1986)	U.S. (Cleveland)	3.0	—	—
Registry based	Chavez et al. (1988)	U.S. (1980-1986)			
		Native Americans	2.9	—	—
		African Americans	0.6	—	—
		Caucasians	0.09	—	—
		Hispanics	0.08	—	—
		Asians	0.03	—	—
Registry based	CDC (1993a)	U.S. (1979-1992)	0.2	—	—
Registry based	CDC (1993b)	U.S. (1992)	0.37	—	—
Population based	May et al. (1983)	SW Native Americans (1969-1982)	2.0	1.1	3.1
		SW Native Americans (1978-1982)	4.2	1.5	5.7
Population based	Asante and Nelms-Matzke (1985)	Native Canadians—British Columbia	—	—	25.0
		Native Canadians—Yukon	—	—	46.0
Population based	Robinson et al. (1987)	NW Canada Indians	120.0	69.0	189.0
Population based	Duimstra et al. (1993)	Plains Indians	3.9-8.5	—	—

NOTE: NW = northwestern; SW = southwestern.

[a]Total reported diagnosed or diagnosable alcohol-related birth defects include those referred to as FAS and ARBD (or FAE).

same study, Hanson et al. found several other infants who were born to mothers with substantial drinking histories and who had some strong FAS features. The rate of possible alcohol-related effects was then 4.6 per 1,000, yielding a total diagnosable alcohol-related abnormality rate of 5.9 for Seattle (calculated from Hanson et al., 1978).

In Boston, two studies yielded FAS incidence rates ranging from 0.6 per 1,000 (Hingson et al., 1982) to 3.1 per 1,000 (Ouellette et al., 1977). In Cleveland, two studies produced estimates of FAS incidence rates ranging from 0.6 per 1,000 (Sokol et al., 1980) to 3.0 per 1,000 (Sokol et al., 1986). Other FAS studies conducted in Denver and Loma Linda found no FAS cases (Abel and Sokol, 1987; 1991).

From the clinic-based studies, one can conclude that the prevalence of FAS varies by the prevalence of the problem in the select population served by the hospital or clinic and by the methodology used for case identification and ascertainment. Such studies typically result in numbers that are higher than prevalence estimates derived by using standard surveillance methodologies.

Prospective Epidemiologic Studies of the Effects of Maternal Substance Abuse

While the clinic-based studies described above focus primarily on the incidence of formally diagnosed cases of FAS, ARBD, or ARND, the approach that some other researchers have taken is to record maternal drinking and drug-taking patterns in large samples from clinic and hospital settings. The children of these women are then followed over time to document birth weight, length, head circumference, structural malformations, and other relevant traits. Few, if any, of the offspring of these women have FAS, because so relatively few of the women who would enroll in such a study abuse alcohol at levels that cause FAS. Most of the women in these studies who drink do so in the light to moderate ranges. The problems of interpretation and the implications of these data are discussed in detail in Chapter 8.

Following children longitudinally provides important information that can support our understanding of the range of alcohol teratogenesis. Day et al. (1989, 1990, 1991) published the results of measuring offspring traits at birth, 8 months, and 3 years of age. In these studies, carried out in Pittsburgh, low birth weight, decreased head circumference and length, two or more minor anomalies, and significantly slower growth were found to be present in the children of mothers who consumed an average daily alcohol volume of one or more drinks during pregnancy (Day et al., 1991). Similar findings came from the Cleveland, Seattle, and Detroit longitudinal studies.

These trait studies are important for several reasons. They document a wider range of fetal alcohol damage than FAS alone, and they focus on more singular, individual, and quantifiable traits in the children, which also creates an advantage in sample size. Further, the longitudinal ascertainment of maternal traits (e.g., drinking patterns and health status), and offspring signs of fetal alcohol exposure in a wider population has considerable utility, because some traits (e.g., hyperactivity) may not emerge until several years after birth. The range of outcomes studied and the longitudinal approach can provide valuable information in planning and evaluating comprehensive programs of prevention, because they both broaden the target of prevention (all levels of alcohol-related effects) and provide a greater range of dependent variables to use as outcome measures. This approach is discussed in more detail later in this chapter. The relation between the incidence of FAS and the incidence of these traits associated with prenatal alcohol exposure is not fully understood.

Population-Based Epidemiology Studies

Population-based epidemiologic studies using active case ascertainment can assist in addressing some of the criticisms mentioned above, can provide relevant information on the magnitude of the problem in specific communities, and may be more useful for comprehensive community-based prevention efforts. The four major population-based studies done in the world to date were all carried out almost exclusively in Native American communities in North America. In these population-based studies, active and extensive community outreach is carried out for case finding, and all children in a particular population are screened for any physical features (e.g., dysmorphology or low birth weight), family history, or other background characteristics that might make them candidates for the diagnosis of FAS or ARBD.

Using a population-based outreach network in northwestern Canada, Asante and Nelms-Matzke (1985) estimated the rate of FAS and possible alcohol-related effects at 46 per 1,000 Native Canadian children in the Yukon and 25 per 1,000 in British Columbia. Furthermore, these authors estimated that 51 to 66 percent of all children in special education with learning disorders in the study regions were exposed to alcohol in utero.

Robinson et al. (1987) screened all children less than 19 years of age in a small Native Canadian community noted for its high rates of alcohol consumption. Twenty-two children born to women who used alcohol during pregnancy and were diagnosed with FAS, or what the committee terms partial FAS, were identified, yielding a prevalence of 190 FAS or partial FAS cases per 1,000 children. This is the highest prevalence rate ever recorded anywhere. Interestingly, these 22 children were produced by 14 mothers (fewer than one-third of the mothers in this heavy-drinking community), and in 46 percent of the total pregnancies the mothers were abstainers. Of the verified drinking pregnancies, 40.7 percent of the children were diagnosed as FAS or partial FAS.

In another population-based prevalence study carried out in seven different Native American communities in the southwestern United States by May and colleagues (May and Hymbaugh 1983; May et al., 1983), 115 children were found to have FAS or traits reminiscent of FAS but less severe. The prevalence of FAS or these less complete cases was highly variable among the three different tribal cultural groups involved in the study. The prevalence of FAS among children 0-14 years was 1.6 per 1,000 for Navajo Indians, 2.2 for Pueblo Indians, and 10.7 for two groups of southwestern Native Americans. Overall, the weighted average rate for southwestern Native Americans was 2.0 per 1,000 for FAS and 3.1 per 1,000 for FAS and the less severe manifestations combined. In the most recent birth cohort studied, however, the FAS rate was higher, 4.2 per 1,000 for FAS and 5.7 for FAS and the other manifestations combined. Of more importance for prevention, however, is the fact that a number of maternal and social risk factors were determined in this study. These findings are presented below.

In a study of four North and South Dakota Plains Indian reservations, Duimstra et al. (1993) used low birth weight and a developmental screening test in an outreach, case-finding network to assess the prevalence of FAS. The rate of FAS confirmed by dysmorphology exam was 3.9 per 1,000. When the rate of confirmed cases was projected to all children identified as suspected cases by the outreach network, necessitated by cases lost to follow-up, the estimated rate of FAS rose to 8.5 per 1,000.

The overall significance of these population-based studies is that they may provide more accurate prevalence data and could point the way to more valuable information for comprehensive prevention programs. By not looking only at the prevalence and characteristics of FAS, ARBD, and ARND as presented in various clinics, population-based studies possess the capability of examining a range of social and cultural influences that impact upon the rate of these conditions. Such conditions may be readily amenable to the design of large-scale or intensive preventive efforts. For example, the rate of maternal risk and the characteristics of the social milieu could help define adequate approaches and targets for prevention and the magnitude of effort required. In addition, the programs of awareness and emphasis on intensive and societal-based efforts of case identification are advantages of population-based approaches. FAS needs such an approach if its prevalence is to be accurately estimated.

In the Native American tribes highlighted in the FAS prevalence studies, the drinking pattern is bimodal: a high proportion of the tribe does not drink at all, but among those who do drink there is a high proportion of heavy and abusive drinkers (May, 1994). Many of those young and middle-aged adults who drink do so in large quantities and generally participate in subcultures emphasizing long binges of heavy drinking leading to very high blood alcohol levels over several days. Because many reservations prohibit the sale and possession of alcohol, drinking is pursued outside the mainstream, normal social activities and law, generally in border town communities away from the reservation and its traditional culture and sanctions. Social isolation and the entrenchment of heavy-drinking behavior among some females, through stigmatization, is common in some tribes. This often leads to a high frequency of FAS, ARBD, and ARND births in some tribes and subcultures within them (May et al., 1983). Alcohol is, by far, the major drug of choice among virtually all Native Americans and tribes, with only occasional use of marijuana, inhalants, or solvents among some problem drinkers (see May, 1994).

Issues and Considerations

It appears, as documented above, that the literature on the prevalence and epidemiology of FAS is far from consistent or conclusive. Various studies reporting the occurrence of FAS range from 0.6 to 3 births per 1,000 in most populations, with some communities having much higher rates. Rates in inner cities, for example, are 2.29 per 1,000 versus 0.26 at sites where the population is middle class (Abel, in press). FAS and other diagnosable ARBD or ARND designations may occur on average in as many as 6 per 1,000 births (May et al., 1983). Because only a proportion of mothers who are very heavy drinkers will have children with FAS (Abel, in press), it is vital that researchers do more to study and compare the social and biological characteristics of FAS mothers with those especially heavy drinkers who do not have FAS children. The consistency and, hence, comparability of the FAS prevalence (and overall epidemiologic) methodology need to be improved. Increased understanding of the maternal characteristics and social variables that influence FAS, ARBD, and ARND is also needed.

Other review articles on FAS have raised key issues regarding most of the epidemiologic studies on possible alcohol-related effects (Abel, in press; Abel and Hannigan, in press; Abel and Sokol, 1987, 1991; Russell, 1991). These key issues include methodologies and definitions in case finding and diagnosis; wide variation in the types of populations studied; consistency of data gathered by prospective versus retrospective methods; and improvements in surveillance techniques. In general, it remains difficult to reconcile incidence and prevalence rates between studies.

Role of Epidemiology in Prevention Programs

The major public health planning document of this decade, Healthy People 2000, states that the baseline incidence rate for FAS for the United States is 0.22 per 1,000 births (U.S. Department of Health and Human Services, 1991b). Furthermore, the goal for the year 2000 is to reduce this figure to 0.12. This goal as an absolute number may be unrealistic given the obvious variances in the incidence and prevalence rates for FAS summarized in Table 5-1 and in the three composite estimates by Abel (in press) and Abel and Sokol (1987, 1991), which indicate worldwide variability of rates ranging from 0.33 per 1,000 to 0.97 per 1,000 (Abel, in press). The latest estimate for the United States is 1.95, far greater than the Healthy People 2000 baseline rate of 0.22 per 1,000 (Abel, in press). Many Healthy People 2000 goals were expressed as a percentage of the baseline and some of those baselines were revisited and changed. A goal of 50 percent reduction, which is what the FAS goal approximates if compared to the baseline of 0.22 per 1,0000, seems more reasonable, but only if the baseline is adjusted to more accurately reflect the consensus of the field. As this chapter illustrates, however, there is no consensus about the incidence of FAS except that it is much higher than the Healthy People 2000 baseline rate. Exactly how much higher is not clear. As long as we do not have consistent methods, criteria for assessment, or sufficient understanding of FAS prevalence, targeted prevention goals will be difficult to monitor.

Consistent Diagnosis

FAS may not be well recognized or routinely and consistently documented by many physicians. In one study in Texas, Little et al. (1990) found that the diagnosis of FAS was not made in the medical records of any of the 40 infants born to 38 women who had at least four alcoholic beverages per day. The charts of six of the infants included notations of features of FAS. In follow-up of these offspring, 17 had very poor growth and development records and other possible indicators of FAS, ARBD, or ARND. Conversely, in other locales FAS may be over diagnosed (Aase, 1994; Abel and Sokol, 1987). In some ethnic minority communities, and communities perceived as having alcohol abuse problems, individuals may be more likely to receive the diagnosis when specific case evidence is marginal (Aase, 1994; Chavez et al., 1988).

Chavez et al. (1988) raised several important issues pertaining to differences in prevalence results with respect to ethnicity. They suggested that (1) physicians tend to be more likely to look for particular malformations among particular ethnic groups; (2) minority status may elevate the rates of reporting particular malformations; (3) hospitals participating in the birth defect monitoring program(s) may not be representative of all hospitals; (4) socioeconomic factors cannot be ruled out as important contributions to the burden of ARBD malformations; and (5) many of the malformations may have been associated with genetic and environmental factors. Each of these issues is relevant for both FAS epidemiology studies and comprehensive prevention programs.

Use of Multiple Data Sources

Several recent projects of surveillance and prevalence assessment have utilized multiple data sources and approaches. In Alaska, multiple secondary data sources were used to estimate statewide and ethnic-specific prevalence (Centers for Disease Control, 1993b; Egeland et al., submitted for publication). By using ICD-9 codes; private sector data sources (inpatient and outpatient); education, genetics, and disability program records; and Alaska Native Health Service records, case definitions were used to estimate FAS prevalence and some descriptive epidemiologic characteristics of FAS children and their mothers. As one would expect, results proved to be similar in many ways to various findings from the other methodologies used as described previously. However, by combining several data sources and using a more active case-finding effort, estimates of prevalence may have been more accurate. In addition, using a combination of active and passive surveillance systems indicated a high FAS prevalence rate among Alaska Natives than by an active screening and referral effort alone.

SURVEILLANCE METHODS FOR FETAL ALCOHOL SYNDROME

On a national level, there are two ways to monitor the impact on public health of alcohol use during pregnancy by using surveillance strategies. The two surveillance approaches discussed in this section involve passive and active methodologies. The advantages and disadvantages of each approach are presented here, along with possible solutions to the problems they pose with respect to FAS. Given the stated goal of reducing FAS, much more attention has to be paid to standardization of data collection, whatever the strategy for assessment.

Passive Surveillance

Passive surveillance is the strategy generally used to monitor birth defects (Lynberg and Edmonds, 1992). This strategy simply tallies the number of cases of a defined birth defect or syndrome noted on existing documents, such as medical records, and relates that figure to some population. Review of individual cases is not done. This is the strategy behind the CDC's Birth Defects Monitoring Program, discussed previously, which used hospital discharge data on both live and stillborn newborns to estimate the incidence of FAS at 2 cases per 10,000 between 1979 and 1992, and 3.7 per 10,000 births in 1992 (CDC, 1993a).

Advantages and Disadvantages

The advantage of passive surveillance for FAS is that it is directly comparable with the methodologies used to assess the incidence of other birth defects, allowing a comparison of relative rates. It allows monitoring of secular changes and differences by geographic distribution or sociodemographic status, as well as comparison of the distributions of different kinds of birth defects.

There are several disadvantages to this methodology, however, for the surveillance of FAS. A major problem is the accuracy with which FAS is diagnosed, particularly at birth. This inaccuracy is due to several factors: (1) it is difficult to evaluate central nervous system (CNS) status at birth; (2) many clinicians are not trained to identify FAS; (3) inconsistent criteria are used for case definition; and

(4) clinicians may be reluctant to identify alcohol problems or to label women as having alcohol problems.

Clinicians continue to use, somewhat idiosyncratically, a diverse pattern of traits to diagnose FAS (Clarren and Astley, 1994). There may also be "selective" case finding by physicians who look for particular malformations among some minority groups compared with others (Chavez et al., 1988). Case finding of pregnant substance abusers similarly focuses on women with certain characteristics (e.g., a history of alcohol or drug use noted in their charts, older age, African-American ethnicity, use of tobacco, a history of social or emotional problems). In the absence of these markers, few pregnant women are screened for alcohol or drug use, and about 50 percent of all relevant cases may be missed by clinic staff (Reynolds and Day, unpublished data). A similar problem may likewise affect detection of FAS.

In addition, the characteristics that are prominent in FAS and used for diagnosis may differ by age. A survey reported by Clarren and Astley (1994) demonstrated that while clinicians consider microcephaly and growth retardation to be important parameters in newborns and infants, in older children they are more likely to consider microcephaly in conjunction with behavioral problems as pathognomonic. A solution would be to use the standardized criteria for diagnosis presented in Chapter 4 of this report.

Possible Solutions

Passive surveillance as used currently can be improved for FAS surveillance. Improvements could be made directly by improving passive surveillance of FAS or indirectly by using proxy indicators of FAS.

Direct Measures   Clinicians can be educated to better recognize FAS. However, it is still likely that biased reporting will continue to occur, given the negative labeling associated with alcohol involvement. It may be difficult to determine accurately the incidence of FAS at birth, particularly in environments where clinicians are not well trained, not sensitive to or willing to report the use of alcohol among pregnant women, or not willing to use standardized diagnostic criteria. Providing a confidential reporting mechanism, separate from the medical record or birth certificate, would reduce this bias. Even in the presence of these improvements, however, correct ascertainment of the rate of FAS at birth remains problematic due to the difficulty in assessing CNS or neurobehavioral abnormalities at this age.

Indirect Indicators   An alternative to monitoring the incidence of FAS at birth is to develop surveillance criteria that would identify a group of newborns with a high probability of having FAS, for example, newborns with birth weights below 2 standard deviations for gestational age. Criteria such as birth weight that are

TABLE 5-2 Predictability of Fetal Alcohol Syndrome Based on Surveillance Criteria

	Head Circumference <10th Percentile and One Facial Anomaly (N = 29)	All Remaining Subjects (N = 713)
Average daily volume (ADV), first trimester	1.37	0.57
ADV third trimester	1.28	0.10
IQ score at age 6	85.5	95.9
Weight at age 6 (kg)	20.9	23.2
Height at age 6 (cm)	113.8	119.5
Head circumference at age 6 (mm)	513.4	521.2

NOTE: All comparisons are significant at $P < 0.001$.

SOURCE: Reynolds and Day, unpublished data.

routinely recognized, measured, and noted in the medical record are not subject to clinical judgment. This strategy was adopted in a study of four American Indian communities where the investigators selected a group of children who had a birth weight of less than 3,000 grams. These children were referred for evaluation for FAS if they had poor performance on a developmental screening test or if they had a head circumference below the 10th percentile; 4 out of 24 suspected cases were confirmed as FAS (Duimstra et al., 1993).

An example of data analyzed for indirect or proxy indicators of FAS is presented in Table 5-2. The data in this table are from the Maternal Health Practices and Child Development Project, an ongoing assessment of the long-term effects of substance use during pregnancy. This is a prospective epidemiologic study of pregnancy outcomes, and one of few that have followed a cohort from early pregnancy up to the child's tenth year. The women selected for this study represent the entire spectrum of alcohol use, although the majority were moderate drinkers and moderate users of other substances. They were interviewed for alcohol use in their fourth and seventh prenatal months, and their offspring were assessed at delivery, 8 and 18 months, and 3 and 6 years of age. The cohort used for analysis was 742 mother-child dyads. Although these data were collected as part of a controlled, prospective epidemiologic study, the data used in the example are representative of data that could be gathered passively for a surveillance effort.

Surveillance criteria for proxy indicators of FAS were defined as either head circumference, weight or height at birth less than the 10th percentile, and the presence of at least one facial anomaly. The facial anomalies were selected from the list of facial dysmorphic features that are part of FAS.

Children who had a growth deficit at birth, defined as weight or height or head circumference below the 10th percentile, combined with the presence of at least one facial anomaly, were significantly more likely to have been exposed to alcohol prenatally; had significantly lower weight, height, and head circumference at three and six years; and scored significantly lower on the composite score of the Stanford-Binet Intelligence Scale. It was not possible, in this moderately exposed population, to estimate the incidence of FAS, but the strategy may lend itself to such estimates if the sample size is large enough.

To establish a relationship between the incidence of cases with the surveillance criteria and the occurrence of FAS, however, would require replicated investigations using dysmorphologists trained in the identification of FAS and follow-up of these research cohorts over the first few years to determine the predictability of the surveillance criteria to the diagnosis.

The advantages of a surveillance program using indirect measures or indicators lie primarily in three areas: (1) lower cost, because the criteria are already ascertained and noted in the birth or other record; (2) more accurate measurement of the criteria; and (3) elimination of the problem of negative labeling of women by clinicians.

The disadvantages of this method lie in the general problem of extrapolating from the surveillance criteria to the incidence of FAS and include pervasive problems pertaining to the diagnostic abilities of clinicians. In addition, a decrease in the prevalence of the indirect marker would not necessarily reflect a proportionate decrease in the prevalence of FAS.

In passive surveillance—whether direct or indirect measurement is used—it is important to monitor multiple sources for the detection of cases (e.g., birth and death certificates, Medicaid claims, private pediatric practice case files) because no one source can identify more than a minority of cases (CDC, 1993b).

Active Surveillance for Fetal Alcohol Syndrome

Active surveillance implies direct collection and review of cases using well-defined protocols rather than using data such as medical charts (Lynberg and Edmonds, 1992). Medical charts can be used as source for potential cases, but these cases are reviewed for the purposes of the surveillance effort. The hallmark of these kinds of protocols for FAS is the prospective epidemiologic study of the effects of maternal substance abuse. In this study every case is followed from a predetermined entry point (time A) to a specifically defined end point (time B; e.g., birth). There have been few examples of active surveillance outside the focused research literature. Most of these studies have had small sample sizes; they are far from representative; and the diagnostic criteria are not consistent (see clinic-based studies in Table 5-1). In general, the rates of FAS are higher by an order of magnitude than those estimated from passive surveillance studies (Abel, in press; Abel and Sokol, 1987, 1991; May, in press).

Advantages and Disadvantages

As illustrated above, a comparison of the incidence rates generated by active and passive surveillance demonstrates that active surveillance detects substantially more cases (Klaucke, 1992; May, in press). Moreover, control over data collection also implies control over data quality. Thus, the diagnoses are more likely to be valid and reliable. Because of this, direct and more accurate measurement of the rate of FAS is possible using active surveillance. Population-based active surveillance programs can be tailored to characteristics of the population under study and can be linked more closely with prevention efforts.

The disadvantages of active surveillance are threefold: (1) it is very expensive to collect data from a population large enough to yield representative rates; (2) it is extremely labor intensive; and (3) it is selective, in that only subjects who appear at entry will be assessed. One report noted a tenfold difference in costs between active and passive surveillance (Klaucke, 1992). The large epidemiologic studies that actively studied effects of maternal alcohol abuse were usually centered in large cities and within academic and research facilities. Other more active surveillance programs for FAS occurred in select populations. As a result, the data are likely to be biased and cannot be extrapolated to the general population. Few cases of FAS were identified in the major prospective epidemiologic studies of maternal substance abuse in major U.S. cities (e.g., Seattle, Pittsburgh), because the alcohol exposure generally was low to moderate. The Atlanta study included many women who drank heavily, and many dysmorphic children were identified.

Proxy Measures in an Active Surveillance Program

Just as passive surveillance can be refined by using or including indirect measures that focus on birth weight or some other indicator for case finding, so too can active surveillance for FAS include proxy measures. The approach to proxy measures suggested for passive surveillance could be used, if validated, for active surveillance of FAS. Population-based studies in representative populations could help determine the best proxy measures for an active surveillance program. Alternatively, prevalence of alcohol abuse can be used indirectly to measure or at least approximate the risk of FAS and the success of prevention efforts. This is because FAS has a known cause—alcohol abuse.

Alcohol Abuse Because FAS, by definition, occurs only among offspring of women who abuse alcohol, a logical point for screening would be alcohol abuse. A screen for alcohol abuse would yield a low rate of cases but would identify women who are at high risk of having a baby with FAS, ARBD, or ARND. This type of screening has two advantages: (1) it identifies the population that is at the highest risk of having a child with FAS, and (2) it identifies a population that is unquestionably in need of intervention.

The disadvantages of this approach, however, are numerous: (1) the diagnosis of alcohol abuse is often unreliable, (2) the diagnosis of alcohol abuse is often avoided by clinicians to preclude labeling women, and (3) women may not report symptoms of alcohol abuse. The availability of a biomarker of alcohol exposure could be useful, but none currently exists that could be used in a surveillance program (see Chapter 7). The rate of FAS among the offspring of women who abuse alcohol is not known; the few estimates available are relatively low (Abel, in press; Abel and Sokol, 1987), and the estimates show a varying rate by birth order (Abel, 1988). Thus, prescreening for alcohol abuse to estimate FAS is problematic.

Drinking Practices   Similar problems can be seen when we consider measuring drinking or heavy drinking during pregnancy, although this is an attractive option, given the opportunities it would present for prevention and intervention. However, measuring drinking or heavy drinking is time intensive and remains an effort that few clinicians are trained or willing to make. Drinking, particularly heavy drinking during pregnancy, is a stigmatized behavior; it is likely to be underreported by women and reported in a biased fashion by clinicians. Moreover, we do not know how "heavy" heavy drinking must be to result in FAS, ARBD, or ARND and we may never be able to arrive at a consensus because of the numerous other social, personal, and biological factors that interact with alcohol consumption to produce FAS, ARBD, and ARND (Abel and Hannigan, in press).

Feasibility of Surveillance

Surveillance of FAS can be accomplished by actively seeking or ascertaining cases of FAS or by establishing surveillance criteria for proxy indicators of FAS and actively ascertaining the incidence or prevalence of cases that meet those criteria. Some suggestions for doing this have been described above. Given the limitations of passive surveillance for FAS, it is possibly more efficient to actively ascertain the incidence or prevalence of cases that meet surveillance criteria for proxy indications and then estimate the rate of FAS. This would require research to validate the criteria, to establish the accuracy of their measurement and reporting, and to determine an appropriate estimation (or "conversion") factor. Population-based epidemiologic studies can be very useful as part of an active surveillance effort. Given the inadequacy of passive surveillance for estimating the magnitude nationally of the FAS problem, for indicating success or failure of prevention efforts, and for identifying FAS children and families in need of clinical, social, and educational services, other approaches need to considered, expanded, and validated.

CONCLUSIONS AND RECOMMENDATIONS

The committee concludes that FAS, ARND, and ARBD are a completely preventable set of birth defects and neurodevelopmental abnormalities and that FAS is arguably the most common known nongenetic cause of mental retardation. Further, ARND and ARBD are reported to occur even more frequently than FAS. Thus, the results of heavy prenatal alcohol exposure constitute a major public health concern. The committee endorses the efforts of the Centers for Disease Control and Prevention to move away from passive surveillance methods, which have been unsuccessful in defining the magnitude of this problem, but recognizes that no national baseline is available to judge the impact of public health and other preventive interventions. The committee encourages CDC's new efforts to implement active surveillance strategies in state- and university-based surveys. However, to address the lack of baseline data and the wide variation of prevalence estimates for subpopulations, including ethnic minorities, the committee recommends that

- an interagency plan be developed for a national survey to estimate the prevalence and incidence of FAS, ARND, and ARBD, which could utilize active surveillance techniques (direct or indirect);
- prevalence surveys of FAS, ARND, and ARBD be repeated at periodic intervals;
- data on prevalence of FAS, ARND, and ARBD be integrated with data on the drinking behavior of pregnant women to improve risk assessment for these disorders;
- improved data collection and surveillance be implemented to identify specifically children with FAS, ARND, and ARBD in various social and educational environments (e.g., maternal and child health block grant programs, Head Start programs, and Early Intervention and Special Education Services); and
- when active surveillance strategies are employed that identify children with FAS, ARND, or ARBD, appropriate linkages should be in place among agencies and local clinics to facilitate treatment.

REFERENCES

Aase JM. Clinical recognition of FAS: Difficulties of detection and diagnosis. Alcohol Health & Research World 1994; 18:5-9.

Abel EL. Commentary: Fetal alcohol syndrome in families. Neurotoxicology and Teratology 1988; 10:12.

Abel EL. An update on incidence of FAS: FAS is not an equal opportunity birth defect. Neurotoxicology and Teratology, in press.

Abel EL, Hannigan JH. Maternal risk factors in fetal alcohol syndrome: Provocative and permissive influences. Neurotoxicology and Teratology, in press.

Abel EL, Sokol RJ. Incidence of fetal alcohol syndrome and economic impact of FAS-related anomalies. Drug and Alcohol Dependence 1987; 19:51-70.

Abel EL, Sokol RJ. A revised conservative estimate of the incidence of FAS and its economic impact. Alcoholism: Clinical and Experimental Research 1991; 15:514-524.

Asante KO, Nelms-Matzke J. Survey of children with chronic handicaps and fetal alcohol syndrome in the Yukon and Northwest B. C. Ottawa. Health and Welfare Canada (unpublished report) 1985.

Beauchamp D. Beyond Alcoholism: Alcohol and Public Health Policy. Philadelphia: Temple University Press, 1980.

Centers for Disease Control. Fetal alcohol syndrome—United States, 1979-1992. Morbidity and Mortality Weekly Report 1993a; 42:339-341.

Centers for Disease Control. Linking multiple data sources in fetal alcohol syndrome surveillance—Alaska. Morbidity and Mortality Weekly Report 1993b; 42:312-314.

Centers for Disease Control and Prevention. Update: Trends in fetal alcohol syndrome—United States, 1979-1993. Morbidity and Mortality Weekly Report 1995a;44:249-251.

Centers for Disease Control and Prevention. Birth certificates as a source for fetal alcohol syndrome case ascertainment—Georgia, 1989-1992. Morbidity and Mortality Weekly Report 1995b; 44:251-253.

Chavez GF, Cordero JF, Becerra JE. Leading major congenital malformations among minority groups in the United States, 1981-1986. Morbidity and Mortality Weekly Report 1988; 37:17-24.

Clarren S., Astley S. Quoted in the Summary Report of the RSA/CDC/NIAAA FAS Data Collaboration Meeting. Atlanta, Georgia, March 17-18, 1994.

Day NL, Jasperse D, Richardson F, Robles N, Sambamoorthis U, Taylor P et al. Prenatal exposure to alcohol: Effect on infant growth and morphologic characteristics. Pediatrics 1989; 84:536-541.

Day NL, Richardson G, Robles N, Sambamoorthis U, Taylor P, Scher M et al. Effect of prenatal alcohol exposure on growth and morphology of offspring at 8 months of age. Pediatrics 1990; 85:748-752.

Day NL, Robles N, Richardson G, Geva D, Taylor P, Scher M et al. The effects of prenatal alcohol use in the growth of children at three years of age. Alcoholism: Clinical and Experimental Research 1991; 15:67-71.

Dehaene P, Crepin G, Delahousse F, Querleu D, Walbaum R, Titian M et al. Aspects epidemiologiques du syndrome d'alcoolisme foetal. La Nouvelle Presse Medicale 1981; 10:2639-2643.

Dehaene P, Samaille-Villette C, Bordaiger-Fasquelle P, Subtel D, Delahouse G, Crepin G. Diagnostic et prevalence du syndrome d'alcoolisme foetal en maternite. La Presse Medicale 1991; 20:1002.

Dehaene P, Samaille-Villette C, Crepin G, Walbaum R, DeRoubaix P, Blanc-Garin A. Le syndrome d'alcoolisme foetal dan le Nord de la France. La Revue de l'Alcoolisme 1977; 23:145-158.

Duimstra D, Johnson C, Kutsch C, Wang B, Zentner M, Kellerman S et al. A fetal alcohol syndrome surveillance pilot project in American Indian communities in the Northern Plains. Public Health Reports 1993; 108:225-229.

Egeland GM, Perham-Hester KA, Gessner BD, Ingle D, Berner J, Middaugh JP. Fetal alcohol syndrome in Alaska. Submitted for publication.

Hanson JW, Streissguth AP, Smith DW. The effects of moderate alcohol consumption during pregnancy on fetal growth and morphogenesis. Journal of Pediatrics 1978; 92:457-460.

Hingson R, Alpert JJ, Day N, Dooling E, Kayne H, Morelock S et al. Effects of maternal drinking and marijuana use on fetal growth and development. Pediatrics 1982; 70:539-546.

Hingson R, Scotch N, Goldman E. Impact of the "Rand Report" on alcoholics, treatment personnel and Boston residents. Journal of Studies on Alcohol 1977; 38:2065-2076.

Klaucke D. Evaluating public health surveillance systems. Public Health Surveillance. W. Halperin and E. Baker (eds.) New York: Van Nostrand Reinhold, 1992:26-41.

Little BB, Snell LM, Rosenfeld CR, Gilstrap LCI, Gant NF. Failure to recognize fetal alcohol syndrome in newborn infants. American Journal of Disease in Children 1990; 144:1142-1146.

Lynberg MC, Edmonds LD. Surveillance of Birth Defects in Public Health Surveillance. William Halperin and Edward L. Baker, Jr. (eds.); Richard R. Monson (consulting ed.). New York: Van Nostrand Reinhold, 1992.

May PA. The epidemiology of alcohol abuse among American Indians: The mythical and real properties. Journal of American Indian Culture 1994; 18:121-143.

May PA. Research issues in the prevention of fetal alcohol syndrome (FAS) and alcohol-related birth defects (ARBD). Prevention Research on Women and Alcohol. E. Taylor, J. Howard, P. Mail, M. Hilton (eds.). Washington, DC: U.S. Government Printing Office, in press.

May PA, Hymbaugh KJ. A pilot project on fetal alcohol syndrome among American Indians. Alcohol Health & Research World 1983; 7:3-9.

May PA, Hymbaugh KJ, Aase JM, Samet JM. Epidemiology of fetal alcohol syndrome among American Indians of the Southwest. Social Biology 1983; 30:374-387.

Olegard R, Sabvel KG, Aronsson J, Sandin B, Johnsson PR, Carlsson C et al. Effects on the child of alcohol abuse during pregnancy: Retrospective and prospective studies. Acta Paediatrica Scandinavia 1979; 275 (Supplement):112-121.

Ouellette EM, Rosett JL, Rosman NP, Weiner L. Adverse effects on offspring of maternal alcohol abuse during pregnancy. New England Journal of Medicine 1977; 297:528-530.

Reynolds M, Day N. Maternal Health Practices and Child Development Project. Unpublished data 1995.

Robinson GC, Conry JL, Conry RF. Clinical profile and prevalence of fetal alcohol syndrome in an isolated community in British Columbia. Canadian Medical Association Journal 1987; 137:203-207.

Russell M. Clinical implications of recent research on the fetal alcohol syndrome. Bulletin of the New York Academy of Medicine 1991; 67:207-222.

Sokol RJ, Ager J, Martier S, Debanne S, Ernhart C, Kuzma J. Significant determinants of susceptibility to alcohol teratogenicity. Annals of the National Academy of Medical Sciences 1986; 477:87-102.

Sokol RJ, Miller SI, Reed G. Alcohol abuse during pregnancy: An epidemiological study. Alcoholism: Clinical and Experimental Research 1980; 4:135-145.

U.S. Department of Health and Human Services. The International Classification of Diseases, 9th Revision, Clinical Modification, ICD-9-CM, Fourth Edition, Vol. 1 Washington, D.C.: U.S. Department of Health and Human Services, 1991a.

U.S. Department of Health and Human Services. Healthy People 2000:National Health Promotion and Disease Prevention Objectives. Rockville, Maryland: U.S. Department of Health and Human Services, 1991b.

6

Epidemiology of Women's Drinking

Publicity about FAS has undoubtedly increased concern about women's drinking and vice versa. However, these two major areas of research have remained relatively isolated from one another. Studies of FAS have primarily addressed biomedical and clinical concerns: offspring characteristics and diagnosis, mechanisms of alcohol effects, dose-response relationships, and effects of prevention efforts in clinical and community settings. FAS-oriented research on pregnant women who drink has focused primarily on measuring alcohol consumption and on identifying women at risk for giving birth to children with FAS, ARBD, or ARND because of their alcohol abuse. Much of this research, however, has paid relatively little attention to psychological and social determinants of maternal drinking behavior. Although surveillance studies have monitored trends in alcohol consumption among women of childbearing age (e.g., the Behavioral Risk Factors Surveys of the Centers for Disease Control and Prevention [CDC]), such surveys are restricted for the most part to assessing a few demographic characteristics, and most have serious limitations in their measurement of alcohol use, reproductive history, and potential predictors of drinking patterns. Studies of pregnant women have rarely attempted to apply findings from recent research on drinking among women in general to better understand influences on *pregnant* women's drinking behavior.

Although researchers have seen changes in drinking patterns during pregnancy over the years, there is no substantive evidence of any change in drinking behavior among women who drink more heavily or abuse alcohol, either in terms of proportions of heavy drinkers at the time of conception or in terms of consumption levels during pregnancy (Hankin et al., 1993a,b). To learn why some pregnant women continue to drink at hazardous levels despite factual knowledge about fetal risks, it is vital to understand the personal and social-environmental risk factors that support maternal drinking (May, in press; Waterson and Murray-Lyon, 1990; Weiner et al., 1989). Related research on women's drinking more generally may provide some answers for understanding the determinants of pregnant women's drinking behavior.

The following sections discuss (1) methodological considerations, (2) definitions and patterns of drinking among women, and (3) needed research on pregnant women's drinking.

METHODOLOGIC CONSIDERATIONS

Conceptualizing and measuring factors that increase the likelihood of drinking among pregnant women represent a complex task. These factors are likely to differ (1) for drinking in early pregnancy versus continued drinking throughout pregnancy; (2) for any alcohol use during pregnancy versus heavier consumption during pregnancy; and (3) for alcohol use during pregnancy versus alcohol abuse or dependence. In addition, learning more about factors that influence women of childbearing age to drink and to abuse alcohol could tell us which women are most likely to be drinking at high-risk levels before pregnancy is recognized.

In addition to personal and environmental risk factors that affect maternal drinking behavior, other factors may combine with alcohol either to reduce or to exacerbate fetal risks. For example, the incidence of FAS among "heavy" drinkers, variously defined (see discussion below), ranges widely but has never been found to be more than 40 percent in any study (Abel, in press). FAS is not unlike other teratogens in this regard. Very few, if any, teratogens have "attack rates" of 100%. A better understanding of biological and life-style characteristics associated with variations in fetal risk at comparable levels of maternal alcohol consumption is needed to understand the diversity in fetal outcome and might suggest prevention strategies that could strengthen naturally occurring protection against adverse fetal effects (Faden and Hanna, 1994).

During the past two decades, research on alcohol use in pregnancy has become increasingly international, including studies from the United Kingdom, France, Norway, Sweden, New Zealand, a multinational European collaborative project, and others (e.g., Plant et al., 1993; Tolo and Little, in press; Waterson and Murray-Lyon, 1989, 1990). However, studies abroad have uncertain utility for detecting social influences on drinking during pregnancy in the United States. For example, frequent alcohol consumption during pregnancy was not related to smoking behavior in a recent national study of women in New Zealand (Counsell et al., 1994). This finding diverges from those in most U.S. studies, which usually find drinking in pregnancy to be associated with smoking (Serdula et al., 1991). Because of the questionable relevance of some international data to social risk factors in this country, the present discussion emphasizes studies conducted in the United States.

Studies of Pregnant Women in Clinical Settings

Most of what is known about correlates of drinking during pregnancy come from studies of pregnant women in hospitals and prenatal clinics. Findings from these clinic-based studies have several methodological limitations. Many of these studies have been conducted in settings that serve special or high-risk populations (e.g., inner-city hospitals serving predominantly lower-socioeconomic status [SES] patients). The socioeconomic background, ethnic composition, and locations of these clinical samples may limit the degree to which their findings can be generalized.

An additional shortcoming of current clinic-based studies is that most include relatively small numbers of women who are heavier drinkers, alcohol abusers, or alcohol dependent. Most women drinkers stop or drastically reduce their drinking when pregnant (Serdula et al., 1991). In the University of Pittsburgh's Maternal Health Practices and Child Development (MHPCD) Project, for example, only 4.6 percent of women reported drinking an average of one drink per day by the end of the third trimester of pregnancy, compared with 44 percent reporting one or more drinks per day before pregnancy (Day et al., 1993). While this striking reduction in alcohol consumption during pregnancy may reduce fetal risk, the small numbers of heavier drinkers in most clinic-based studies, and the limited variation in drinking levels among pregnant women who do drink, reduce the statistical "power" to detect predictors of maternal drinking behavior.

A final limitation of many clinic-based studies is that most have measured only a few demographic characteristics as predictors of maternal drinking and its effects. Few studies of drinking during pregnancy assess personality or social-environmental variables associated with drinking. Factors such as depression, low self-esteem, family history of alcoholism, partner drinking, sexual dysfunction, and sexual abuse or other violent victimization have related to drinking in studies of women in general (e.g., Miller et al., 1993; Wilsnack, in press, a,b) and may be predictive of drinking behavior for pregnant women as well. Also largely unexplored are the dietary behaviors that may affect biological susceptibilities to alcohol's effects (e.g., intake of antioxidants) (Abel and Hannigan, in press). Learning more about such personal, social, and biological risk factors for drinking in pregnancy might permit prevention efforts to be targeted more effectively to specific maternal risk drinkers.

Studies of Pregnant Women in the General Population

One way to overcome the limitations of smaller and less representative clinical samples is to survey large representative samples of pregnant women in the general population. Because only a small percentage of women are pregnant at any point, only general population surveys with very large samples will allow reliable analysis of drinking correlates among women pregnant at the time of the survey. Some very large national data sets are available that include information on women's drinking behavior, drinking-related problems, and a variety of other health behaviors (see NIAAA, 1994). Unfortunately, many of the largest national alcohol and health surveys (some with samples of more than 40,000 respondents) have not included questions about respondents' pregnancy status. Some examples of large national data sets that do include information about pregnancy status are described in Box 6-1.

Other Issues

Large general population samples of pregnant women will not solve all the problems of measuring alcohol use during pregnancy. Underreporting of alcohol consumption appears to vary by stage of pregnancy (e.g., Day et al., 1993) and may be substantial: recent drug studies suggest that substance use reported in pregnancy may need an upward correction by a factor of three or more (Dicker and Leighton, 1994). It should be borne in mind that reasons for underreporting of illegal substance use may be different from reasons for underreporting alcohol use, and the correction factors may be different. Underreporting obviously complicates the task of estimating dose-response relationships. Valid, sensitive, and specific measures of alcohol exposure in women and in pregnant women, when available, could be very useful. See Chapter 7 for more discussion of potential markers. In addition, it is uncertain whether underreporting may vary systematically (e.g., with drinking levels, education and SES, prenatal care, and other health and life-style variables) in ways that may bias observed relationships between alcohol use during pregnancy and possible risk or protective factors.

Efforts to identify high-risk demographic categories for drinking during pregnancy may overlook heterogeneity within such categories. Thus, in the United States, both clinic-based studies (Day et al., 1993) and population-based surveys (Faden et al., 1994) find bimodal distributions of drinking within several ethnic minority groups. For example, both abstention rates and rates of heavier drinking tend to be higher among pregnant African Americans, Native Americans, and Native Canadians. Heterogeneity is also characteristic of incidence rates for FAS in different communities, with FAS occurring more often in areas characterized by poverty compared with more affluent settings or in areas with cultural lifestyles that include heavy drinking compared to the general population (Abel, in press).

FETAL ALCOHOL SYNDROME

BOX 6-1
Some Survey Sources of Data on
Drinking by Pregnant Women

National Longitudinal Survey of Youth (NLSY)

The NLSY is a multistage, stratified area probability sample designed to be representative of noninstitutionalized American youth aged 14-21 as of January 1, 1979. Supplemental samples included ethnic minority and economically disadvantaged youth, and youth aged 17-21 serving in the military. A total of 12,686 respondents were sampled and followed annually. Questions about alcohol use and alcohol problems were included in most annual surveys in the 1980s. Between 1979 and 1986, 3,322 female respondents had 5,876 live-born children (Faden and Hanna, 1994).

National Maternal and Infant Health Interview Survey (NMIHS), 1988-1991

The NMIHS was a mailed, follow-back survey of a nationally representative sample of 11,000 women who had a live birth during 1988; 4,000 women who had a late fetal death; and 6,000 women who had an infant death in 1988. A longitudinal follow-up of subsamples of each group was conducted in 1991. Detailed information was gathered on drinking behavior before and during pregnancy, demographic characteristics, tobacco and marijuana use, and prenatal and postnatal care.

CDC Behavioral Risk Factors Surveillance Surveys (BRFSS)

BRFSS telephone surveys, coordinated by the CDC, are conducted by most states (48 and the District of Columbia in 1991). The surveys are designed to obtain state-specific prevalence estimates of health behaviors associated with leading causes of death and chronic disease. Alcohol questions include quantity and frequency of consumption, frequency of consuming five or more drinks on an occasion, and frequency of driving after drinking. Recent surveys have included approximately 50,000 respondents; in the 1991 survey, 1,067 women reported being pregnant at the time of the interview (CDC, 1994).

National Pregnancy and Health Survey, 1994

The National Institute on Drug Abuse conducted a survey to provide national estimates of drug use during pregnancy and demographic information about women who use drugs during pregnancy. Unfortunately, alcohol information from the survey is apparently limited to a single question about any use, with no questions about quantity, frequency, or pattern of alcohol use during pregnancy.

Other U.S. National Data Sets

Examination of a recent directory of national health and alcohol data sets (NIAAA, 1994) reveals several additional U.S. national surveys that have included questions about both drinking behavior and pregnancy history. In some cases (e.g., the 1987 National Health and Nutrition Examination Survey I Epidemiologic Follow-up Studies [NHEFS]), it is unclear whether the sample size (1987 NHEFS $N = 9,998$) would generate large enough numbers of pregnant women for analysis. In the case of two studies specific to pregnancy—the 1980 National Fetal Mortality Survey and the 1980 National Natality Survey—levels of reported alcohol consumption are low, limiting the numbers of moderate and heavier drinkers available for analysis. The largest and most recent national alcohol survey—the 1992 National Longitudinal Alcohol Epidemiologic Study ($N = 42,862$ adults age 18 and older)—does not include questions about pregnancy status.

DEFINITIONS AND PATTERNS OF DRINKING
AMONG U.S. WOMEN

Women in the General Population

Alcohol consumption patterns among women in the general U.S. population provide a context for discussing drinking behavior of pregnant women. Approximately 60 percent of adult women in the United States drink alcohol at least occasionally. Of these, the large majority consume small to moderate amounts of alcohol without adverse social, behavioral, or health consequences. In a 1991 U.S. national survey of 1099 women age 21 and older, 58 percent had consumed alcohol in the past 12 months: 44 percent of the sample were classified as light drinkers (women who reported consuming an average of 0-3 standard drinks per week); 12 percent were classified as moderate drinkers (4-13 drinks per week); and 3 percent were classified as heavy drinkers (14 or more drinks per week) (Wilsnack et al., 1994). Rates of drinking and heavy drinking tend to be highest among young women and to decline steadily with age. In the 1991 national survey, for example, 73 percent of women in their twenties and 69 percent of women in their thirties had consumed alcohol in the past 12 months; 4 percent of women in their twenties and thirties reported consuming at least 14 drinks per week. Despite concerns about an "epidemic" of alcohol problems in women in the 1970s and 1980s (e.g., Fillmore, 1984), rates of drinking and heavy drinking have been relatively stable among both women and men, with modest increases in the 1970s and modest declines since the early 1980s (Midanik and Clark, 1994; Williams and DeBakey, 1992; Wilsnack et al., 1994).

Pregnant Women

Available data indicate substantially lower rates of both drinking and heavier drinking among pregnant women, relative to nonpregnant women of childbearing age. For example, less than 25 percent of pregnant women reported *any* use of alcohol in the 1989 National Longitudinal Survey of Youth (20 percent); the 1988 National Maternal and Infant Health Survey (NMIHS; 21 percent); the 1991 CDC Behavioral Risk Factors Surveillance Survey (BRFSS; 14 percent); and the 1994 National Institute on Drug Abuse (NIDA) Pregnancy and Health Survey (19 percent). By comparison, the NIDA survey estimates that 20 percent of pregnant woman smoked, 5.5 percent used any illicit drugs, 0.9 percent used crack cocaine, and 10 percent used psychotherapeutics for medically-indicated conditions. Trend data suggest a significant decline in prenatal alcohol use during the past decade. For example, annual BRFSS surveys conducted in 21 states between 1985 and 1988 found that pregnant women's self-reports of any alcohol consumption in the past month declined from 32 percent to 20 percent over the study period (Serdula et al., 1991).

The dramatic reduction in most women's alcohol consumption when they become pregnant affects how drinking levels are defined in studies of drinking and pregnancy. As just described, use of a standard general population definition of "heavy drinking" (e.g., the criterion of 14 or more drinks per week reached by 4 percent of women age 21-40 in the 1991 U.S. BRFSS survey) would identify fewer than 0.5 percent of pregnant women in most FAS-related studies. This downward shift in drinking distributions in pregnancy helps explain why alcohol and pregnancy research typically uses lower cutoffs for moderate and heavy drinking (e.g., one or more standard drinks per day to define heavy drinking) than do general population surveys (which in turn use lower cutoffs than many popular images of "heavy" drinking). Precise specification of consumption levels considered as "moderate" or "heavy" can aid both professionals and the general public in understanding the implications of scientific research on the fetal effects of maternal alcohol consumption.

Although definitions of heavy drinking vary across studies, rates tend to be very low regardless of the definition used. For example, data from the 1991 BRFSS survey shows that 2 percent of all women of child-bearing age but only 0.3 percent of pregnant women reported drinking 60 or more drinks during the preceding month and 21 percent of all women of child-bearing age but only 1.3 percent of pregnant women reported binge drinking (five or more drinks on at least one occasion) during the preceding month (Centers for Disease Control and Prevention, 1994). Although 45 percent of the respondents to the 1988 NMIHS survey reported drinking alcohol during the 3 months before they learned of their pregnancy, 21 percent drank after they learned of their pregnancy, 0.6 percent had six or more drinks per week during pregnancy, and 0.2 percent reported average consumption of two or more drinks per day (Centers for Disease Control and Prevention, 1995). In four states collaborating in a Pregnancy Risk Assessment Monitoring System (PRAMS) in 1988-1989, proportions of pregnant women reporting consumption of 14 or more drinks per week ranged from 0.03 percent to 0.13 percent (Bruce et al., 1993). Although these percentages are small in *relative* terms, the large *absolute numbers* of women who continue to engage in heavy and hazardous drinking throughout pregnancy make it imperative to understand the personal and social factors that make women more likely to continue drinking heavily during pregnancy.   .

Correlates of Drinking in Pregnancy

Correlates of drinking in early pregnancy are similar to those for women of childbearing age in general. This is because women often don't know they are pregnant until a month or two has passed. They therefore engage in their customary drinking habits early in pregnancy. The correlates include being Caucasian, older, and more educated (Streissguth et al., 1991). Although a number of studies compare correlates of drinking behavior in earlier versus later stages of pregnancy, little attention has been given to correlates of first-trimester drinking before and after pregnancy is confirmed: Do women who change their drinking patterns immediately upon learning of, or suspecting, pregnancy differ from women who change their drinking behavior more gradually?

Older pregnant women in some national samples were more likely than younger pregnant women to report drinking (Centers for Disease Control and Prevention, 1995; National Institute on Drug Abuse, 1994; Serdula et al., 1991), but the percentage of women over 25 years of age who drank during pregnancy has decreased between 1985 and 1988 to that of women 18 to 24 years of age. The NMIHS, a survey of women who gave birth in 1988, suggests that women who drink while pregnant are more likely to be white, more educated, of a higher income level, married, or smokers (Centers for Disease Control and Prevention, 1995). That same survey showed that heavy drinking while pregnant was more prevalent among women who were more than 35 years of age, non-white, and unmarried. Other factors associated with heavy drinking in these pregnant women were low annual household income and no prenatal care. Other studies tend to support that general profile of pregnant women who drink (Day et al., 1993; Waterson and Murray-Lyon, 1990). Correlates of continued drinking during pregnancy despite information on the risks and referral for intervention include onset of drinking behaviors at a young age, heavy drinking on the part of parents and siblings (especially female relatives), evidence of alcohol-related physical problems, and qualifying for a diagnosis of alcohol dependence (Smith et al., 1987).

The list of correlates of drinking during pregnancy is quite short when compared with the broader range of predictors that have been identified or suggested for drinking among women in general. These predictors include familial and genetic factors (e.g., maternal or paternal alcoholism); demographic and social role variables (e.g., lack of social roles, nontraditional employment, unemployment, cohabitation, divorce or separation); individual psychological factors (e.g., depression, anxiety, low self-esteem, eating disorders); relationship variables (e.g., partner's drinking, relationship conflict/violence, sexual dysfunction), physical and sexual victimization; and drinking contexts (including drinking behavior of coworkers and significant others) (see Galanter et al., in press; Gomberg and Nirenberg, 1993; Wilsnack, in press, a,b).

NEEDED RESEARCH ON PREGNANT WOMEN'S DRINKING

Increased Coordination of Research on FAS and Women's Drinking

Increased communication between FAS researchers and researchers studying women's drinking more generally might give FAS researchers a broader framework for detecting risk factors that affect drinking during pregnancy, which in turn might suggest new approaches to FAS prevention. For example, if depression or anxiety strongly predicted continued drinking in pregnancy, this might suggest evaluating psychotherapeutic interventions for these conditions. Associations between pregnant women's heavy drinking and their partners' heavy alcohol or drug use (Abel, 1983), or violent behavior by their partners, might suggest interpersonal and environmental approaches for reducing these women's alcohol use (Masis and May, 1991; Weiner et al., 1989).

Increased Secondary Analysis of National Health and Alcohol Use Surveys

Several large national data sets that contain information on both alcohol use and reproductive history may be of value for examining correlates of drinking and heavy drinking among women of childbearing age, and correlates of drinking and heavy drinking among women pregnant at the time of the surveys. In addition to demographic characteristics, creative use of other information available in the data sets may allow the discovery of additional risk factors even without new data collection. Results of such secondary analyses could then be applied to the design of pregnancy-specific epidemiologic research. National surveys that lack adequate measures of either pregnancy status or alcohol use, however, cannot be employed for these purposes. Inclusion of standard questions about alcohol use and reproductive history in future large national health surveys, as appropriate, will pay high dividends in increased knowledge about drinking during pregnancy, its causes, and its effects. It could also be of benefit if national health surveys, as appropriate, included carefully selected variables (potential risk factors) that have shown strong and consistent relationships to women's drinking and drinking problems in other research.

Inclusion of Ethnic and Other Subgroup Populations in Studies of Drinking in Pregnancy

The large differences in FAS prevalence rates across several racial and ethnic groups are discussed elsewhere in this chapter (see also Abel, in press). In addition to biological and environmental factors that may contribute to these differences in pregnancy outcomes, differences between and within ethnic groups affect pregnant women's drinking behavior in ways that are poorly understood. Culture shapes women's expectations and experiences of both pregnancy and alcohol use (Abel and Hannigan, in press; May et al., 1983). There is a particular need for research on ethnic differences in patterns of alcohol use or nonuse during pregnancy, and on ethnic similarities or differences in women's responses to education and prevention programs designed to reduce the risks of drinking in pregnancy.

Research discussed earlier suggests that a woman's age and socioeconomic status when she becomes pregnant may influence how she uses or abstains from alcohol (Abel and Hannigan, in press). Effective interventions to reduce risks of FAS may require an understanding of age- and status-specific risk factors (e.g., employment experiences) in addition to ethnic and cultural influences. Other potentially important subgroups include unmarried versus married mothers, and women living in heavier-drinking environments (e.g., with a partner who drinks heavily) versus lighter- or nondrinking environments.

Substance-Specific Versus Multiple-Substance Risk Factors

Although much of this discussion has focused on women's use of alcohol during pregnancy, many women who drink during pregnancy abuse other licit and illicit substances as well (Hingson et al., 1982; Serdula et al., 1991; Waterson and Murray-Lyon, 1989). Comparative data on women's use of various substances in combination with alcohol during pregnancy (e.g., Day et al., 1993) are scarce and should be obtained for larger and more representative samples. Studies designed to learn whether risk and protective factors are the same or different for different substances (e.g., alcohol, tobacco, marijuana), and for various specific combinations of substances, could have important implications for the development of single-substance versus multiple-substance approaches to education and prevention.

CONCLUSIONS AND RECOMMENDATIONS

The committee concludes that clinic-based studies of pregnant women have included only a limited range of biologic and psychosocial variables as possible risk factors for drinking in pregnancy. Furthermore, most large national health surveys contain inadequate data on women's drinking or pregnancy status. The lack of such data severely limits the ability to predict which women are most likely to engage in high-risk drinking during pregnancy or to give birth to a child with FAS, ARND, or ARBD. Therefore, the committee recommends special attention to the following research questions and issues:

• expand studies of pregnant women, where possible, to include measurement of psychological, social-environmental, dietary, and other factors that may influence women's drinking behavior or fetal outcome;
• inclusion of questions regarding alcohol consumption and pregnancy status in appropriate future national health surveys;
• standardization of questions added to health surveys regarding the quantity, frequency, and variability of alcohol consumption so as to permit comparisons across multiple surveys;
• studies focused on protective factors that may decrease women's drinking or prevent fetal injury from alcohol consumption;

• studies of women who have successfully stopped heavy or abusive drinking; and

• continued and increased epidemiological study of women's drinking patterns, including efforts to maximize the validity of self-report measures, efforts which should include the use, when possible and appropriate, of a biomarker for alcohol exposure.

REFERENCES

Abel EL. Marihuana, Tobacco, Alcohol, and Reproduction. Boca Raton, FL: CRC Press, 1983.

Abel EL. An update on incidence of FAS: FAS is not an equal opportunity birth defect. Neurotoxicology and Teratology, in press.

Abel EL, Hannigan JH. Maternal risk factors in fetal alcohol syndrome: Provocative and permissive influences. Neurotoxicology and Teratology, in press.

Bruce FC, Adams MM, Shulman HB, Martin ML. Alcohol use before and during pregnancy. American Journal of Preventive Medicine 1993; 9:267-273.

Centers for Disease Control and Prevention. Frequent alcohol consumption among women of childbearing age—Behavioral risk factor surveillance system, 1991. Journal of the American Medical Association 1994; 271:1820-1821.

Centers for Disease Control and Prevention. Sociodemographic and behavioral characteristics associated with alcohol consumption during pregnancy—United States, 1988. Morbidity and Mortality Weekly Report 1995; 44:261-264.

Counsell AM, Smale PN, Geddis DC. Alcohol consumption by New Zealand women during pregnancy. New Zealand Medical Journal 1994; 107:278-281.

Day NL, Cottreau CM, Richardson GA. The epidemiology of alcohol, marijuana, and cocaine use among women of childbearing age and pregnant women. Clinical Obstetrics and Gynecology 1993; 36:232-245.

Dicker M, Leighton EA. Trends in the US prevalence of drug-using parturient women and drug-affected newborns, 1979 through 1990. American Journal of Public Health 1994; 84:1433-1438.

Faden VB, Graubard BI, Dufour M. Drinking by expectant mothers - What does it mean for their babies? Working paper, Division of Biometry and Epidemiology, National Institute on Alcohol Abuse and Alcoholism, 1994.

Faden VB, Hanna EZ. Alcohol and pregnancy—To drink or not to drink? Paper Presented at the Conference on Psychosocial and Behavioral Factors in Women's Health. American Psychological Association, Washington, DC, 1994.

Fillmore KM. "When angels fall": Women's drinking as cultural preoccupation and as reality. Alcohol problems in women: Antecedents, consequences, and intervention. S. C. Wilsnack and L. J. Beckman (eds.). New York: Guilford Press, 1984.

Galanter M, Begleiter N, Deitrich R, Gallant D, Goodwin D, Gottheil E et al. Recent Developments in Alcoholism. Volume 12: Alcoholism in Women. New York: Plenum, in press.

Gomberg ESL, Nirenberg RD. Women and Substance Abuse. Norwood, New Jersey: Ablex, 1993.

Hankin JR, Firestone IJ, Sloan JJ, Ager JW, Goodman AC, Sokol RJ et al. The impact of the alcohol warning label on drinking during pregnancy. Journal of Public Policy & Marketing 1993a; 12:10-18.

Hankin JR, Sloan JJ, Firestone IJ, Ager JW, Sokol RJ. A time series analysis of the impact of the alcohol warning label on antenatal drinking. Alcoholism: Clinical and Experimental Research 1993b; 17:284-289.

Hingson R, Alpert JJ, Day N, Dooling E, Kayne H, Morelock S et al. Effects of maternal drinking and marijuana use on fetal growth and development. Pediatrics 1982; 70:539-546.

Ihlen BM, Amundsen A, Sande HA, Daae L. Changes in the use of intoxicants after onset of pregnancy. British Journal of Addiction 1990; 85:1627-1631.

Masis KB, May PA. A comprehensive local program for the prevention of fetal alcohol syndrome. Public Health Reports 1991; 106:484-489.

May PA. Research issues in the prevention of fetal alcohol syndrome (FAS) and alcohol-related birth defects (ARBD). Prevention Research on Women and Alcohol. E. Taylor, J. Howard, P. Mail, M. Hilton (eds.). Washington, DC: U.S. Government Printing Office, in press.

May PA, Hymbaugh KJ, Aase JM, Samet JM. Epidemiology of fetal alcohol syndrome among American Indians of the Southwest. Social Biology 1983; 30:374-387.

Midanik LR, Clark WB. The demographic distribution of US drinking patterns in 1990: Description and trends from 1984. American Journal of Public Health 1994; 84:1214-1222.

Miller BA, Downs WR, Testa M. Interrelationships between victimization experiences and women's alcohol use. Journal of Studies on Alcohol 1993; 11 (Supplement):109-117.

National Institute on Alcohol Abuse and Alcoholism. Alcohol Epidemiologic Data Directory, June 1994. Washington, DC: Alcohol Epidemiologic Data System, NIAAA/Cyrus Corporation, 1994.

National Institute on Drug Abuse. NIDA survey examines extent of women's drug use during pregnancy. NIDA Media Advisory. Rockville, MD: NIDA, 1994.

Plant M, Sullivan FM, Guerri C, Abel EL. Alcohol and pregnancy. Health Issues Related to Alcohol Consumption. P. M. Verschuren (ed.). Brussels: International Life Sciences Institute, 1993.

Serdula M, Williamson DF, Kendrick JS, Anda RF, Byers T. Trends in alcohol consumption by pregnant women: 1985 through 1988. Journal of the American Medical Association 1991; 265:876-879.

Smith IE, Lancaster JS, Moss-Wells S, Coles CD, Falek A. Identifying high-risk pregnant drinkers: Biological and behavioral correlates of continuous heavy drinking during pregnancy. Journal of Studies on Alcohol 1987; 48:304-309.

Streissguth AP, Grant TM, Barr HM, Brown ZA, Mayock DE, Ramey SL et al. Cocaine and the use of alcohol and other drugs during pregnancy. American Journal of Obstetrics and Gynecology 1991; 164:1239-1243.

Tolo K, Little RE. The epidemiology of alcohol consumption and pregnancy. Gender and Alcohol. R. W. Wilsnack and S. C. Wilsnack (eds.). New Brunswick, New Jersey: Rutgers Center of Alcohol Studies, in press.

Waterson EJ, Murray-Lyon IM. Alcohol, smoking and pregnancy: Some observations on ethnic minorities in the United Kingdom. British Journal of Addiction 1989; 84:323-325.

Waterson EJ, Murray-Lyon IM. Preventing alcohol related birth damage: A review. Social Science and Medicine 1990; 30:349-364.

Weiner L, Morse BA, Garrido P. FAS/FAE: Focusing prevention on women at risk. International Journal of the Addictions 1989; 24:385-395.

Williams GD, DeBakey SF. Changes in levels of alcohol consumption: United States, 1983-1988. British Journal of Addiction 1992; 87:643-648.

Wilsnack SC. Alcohol Use and Alcohol Problems in Women. Psychology of Women's Health: Progress and Challenges in Research and Application. A. L. Stanton and S. J. Gallant (eds.). Washington, DC: American Psychological Association, in press, a.

Wilsnack SC. Patterns and trends in women's drinking: Recent findings and some implications for prevention. Prevention Research on Women and Alcohol. E. Taylor, J. Howard, P. Mail, M. Hilton (eds.). Washington, DC: U.S. Government Printing Office, in press, b.

Wilsnack SC, Wilsnack RW, Hiller-Sturmhofel S. How women drink: Epidemiology of women's drinking and problem drinking. Alcohol Health & Research World 1994; 18:173-181.

7

Prevention of Fetal Alcohol Syndrome

Fetal Alcohol Syndrome (FAS), alcohol-related birth defects (ARBD), and alcohol-related neurodevelopmental disorder (ARND), result from a complicated set of factors that influence exposure, whether a woman who abuses alcohol becomes pregnant and continues to drink throughout pregnancy, and vulnerability to adverse fetal effects at a given level of exposure. Some of these pose opportunities for prevention, others are impediments. Alcohol is a legal drug consumed by many people, but its abuse carries heavy costs—for the individual and for society—apart from costs associated with FAS. Many people who abuse alcohol do not get the help they need, either because they do not have access to the health care or social services system or because some health care or social services professionals are uncomfortable talking with patients about substance abuse problems. Finally, the use and abuse of alcohol have long been centered in emotional and moral debate. Women who abuse alcohol or other substances are particularly stigmatized.

The complicated interrelation among alcohol, women, pregnancy, the woman's spouse or other significant partner and community, and the health care profession means that the prevention of FAS, ARBD, and ARND requires a comprehensive program encompassing a variety of approaches. Because alcohol abuse during pregnancy most likely is associated with a number of different drinking patterns which have various characteristics and etiologies, concepts from cultural, sociological, behavioral, public health, and medical disciplines are relevant to the etiology and prevention of FAS and related conditions.

This chapter discusses prevention efforts aimed at the mother and people with whom she has close personal relationships, and relevant sectors of the community prior to the birth of an affected baby. The next chapter describes prevention efforts that might be aimed at the baby and the family after the child is born to ameliorate the effects of prenatal exposure—that is, efforts aimed at preventing secondary disabilities once a child with FAS, ARBD, or ARND is born. The approach to prevention of FAS, ARBD, and ARND contained in this chapter is conceptually broad and includes treatment and maintenance for those few women who drink heavily during pregnancy. The chapter begins with a general framework for discussing prevention. This is followed by an in-depth description of prevention strategies for women at risk of giving birth to an FAS child.

A PUBLIC HEALTH MODEL OF PREVENTION

The challenge in broad-based prevention is to alter behavior within a variety of settings (Casswell and Gilmore, 1989; Mosher and Jernigan, 1989). Change that occurs in familial, religious, social, economic, judicial, educational, and health care institutions can affect individual and group behavior. Since all social institutions can be potential agents of change (Bloom, 1981), a broad-based approach seems to be most appropriate. A comprehensive FAS prevention program should provide multiple and overlapping levels of reinforcement, incentives, and controls. Most prevention efforts should be aimed at the mother, and to some degree at the father, of the child. Preventing the birth of a child with FAS may involve different actions affecting maternal behavior: broad-based prevention; targeted prevention efforts with the woman, her spouse or other significant partner(s), and additional significant family members; alcohol abuse treatments; contraceptive services; and aftercare.

It is important to note that the committee was charged with discussing what is known from a *research* base about preventing FAS, ARBD, and ARND. There is a wealth of information being generated from communities concerned about the FAS problem. Many of these projects derive from common sense approaches and entail community support, general programs to increase protective factors and decrease risk factors for alcohol abuse, and the like. Reasonable and necessary services are provided to pregnant, substance-abusing women. As with many current health interventions, however, the utility and value of many of these programs as prevention efforts is unknown because of the limited evaluative component of the programs. As this chapter points out, controlled research on the prevention of FAS is scarce. Also, as discussed in greater detail in a subsequent section, it is not clear if these programs are available to, used by, or effective for those women who abuse alcohol in a manner that puts their fetus at risk for FAS, ARBD, or ARND.

The committee found it helpful to think about and analyze the prevention of FAS and related problems within a conceptual framework. Two structures were considered by the committee—the classic framework of primary, secondary, and tertiary prevention and a framework developed by the IOM Committee on Prevention of Mental Disorders (IOM, 1994). In more classical terms, primary prevention refers to a focus on healthy persons and seeks to avoid the onset of disease processes (IOM, 1991). Secondary prevention involves early detection and treatment of persons with early or asymptomatic disease, and tertiary prevention concentrates on arresting the progression of a condition and on preventing or limiting additional impairment. The committee decided to use the latter framework (IOM, 1994), which describes a spectrum of seven levels of intervention, as a more appropriate tool, with some adaptation, to discuss prevention of FAS, ARBD, and ARND. The hallmark of this framework is that one enters into the continuum of interventions in a manner proportional to the certainty and severity of the risk involved. That is, the intervention becomes more specific and intensive as the risk is defined less by general population characteristics and more by individual characteristics.

The model presented was originally described by Gordon (1983, 1987) and subsequently adapted for an IOM committee (IOM, 1994). The model includes a broad spectrum of prevention measures. The model also includes two related components—treatment and maintenance. Prevention activities vary from population-wide programs to efforts aimed at an individual at high risk. Prevention is divided into three levels (*universal, selective,* and *indicated*), treatment into two (*case identification* and *standard treatment* for known disorders), and maintenance into two (*compliance with long-term treatment* and *aftercare*). The model developed by the IOM in 1994 required slight modifications for applicability to FAS, but the general concepts remain the same (see Figure 7-1). This will be explained in the next section. The committee to study fetal alcohol syndrome also stresses that core research in fields such as biomedicine, behavioral and social sciences, and epidemiology support, inform, and are vital to research in FAS prevention.

Because significant people in the life of a woman can play a crucial role in encouraging a healthy pregnancy or, unfortunately, encouraging unhealthy practices, the committee took a family-oriented approach to prevention. Clearly, a woman's partner and her community are appropriate targets for prevention interventions and subjects for prevention intervention research. After the birth of an FAS child, there are two targets for intervention—the mother and the child. Each of them is a patient in need of care; each is a target for treatment and maintenance as well as for prevention intervention for the birth of another FAS child. Case identification of FAS, ARBD, and ARND is described in Chapter 4. Treatment and maintenance of the person with FAS are discussed in Chapter 8.

Definitions

Universal prevention attempts to promote the health and well-being of all individuals in society or of a particular community. Universal prevention interventions are those targeted to the general public to or an entire population group

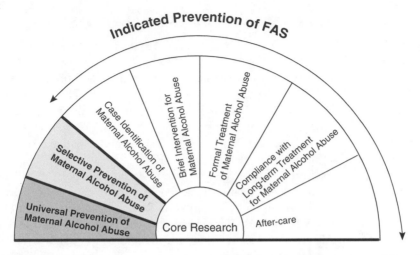

FIGURE 7-1 The intervention spectrum for fetal alcohol syndrome. Adapted from Institute of Medicine (1994).

that has not been identified on the basis of individual risk. The intervention is desirable for everyone in that group. Examples include universal childhood immunizations and water fluoridation.

Selective prevention interventions are targeted to individuals or a subgroup of the population, whose risk of developing the condition is significantly higher than others by virtue of belonging to that subgroup. There is no assessment of individual risk in selective prevention interventions. An example would be routine mammograms for women over 40 to 50 years of age. Another example would be typhoid vaccine for Americans traveling to less developed countries.

Indicated prevention interventions are targeted to high-risk individuals who are identified as having minimal but detectable signs or symptoms foreshadowing a condition or who have biological markers indicating predisposition (IOM, 1994). An example, in contrast to that offered for selective prevention interventions, would be frequent mammograms in a woman who has had breast cancer. Another example is rabies vaccination in someone bitten by a raccoon with unknown rabies status. Special considerations related to FAS necessitated some modification of this definition. That is, although prevention interventions are generally thought of as stopping short of treatment interventions, when thinking about a comprehensive prevention program for FAS, ARBD, and ARND, it is clear that *treatment* of alcohol problems in pregnant women (and their partners) is an appropriate indicated *prevention* intervention for the fetus being carried by the woman, as well as for future pregnancies. In addition, treatment of alcohol problems in the pregnant woman will improve her health and well-being.

UNIVERSAL PREVENTION INTERVENTIONS

Universal prevention interventions are directed to the general public or to an entire population group that has not been identified on the basis of increased risk. Interventions tailored specifically to pregnant women or preconceptional women could be included in this category. Universal prevention could include any activity that generally promotes responsible use of alcohol and discourages irresponsible use of alcohol, or it could be specific to fetal alcohol syndrome. As described later, it is not clear whether these general interventions have had, or could ever have, an impact on FAS, ARBD, or ARND.

General universal prevention strives to ensure that all members of society understand that drinking alcohol can have hazardous consequences, and it promotes and supports positive, broadly shared attitudes and beliefs to protect the individual from harm due to alcohol consumption. The committee focused on FAS, ARBD, and ARND, which are related to consumption of very high levels of alcohol or to extreme patterns of alcohol consumption. They have not reviewed the literature on the health benefits (e.g., cardiovascular) of modest alcohol consumption except to note that there are some data to suggest such benefits for certain populations (Ashley et al., 1994; Fuchs et al., 1995). Moderate alcohol consumption as a substitute for abstinence or light drinking should not be encouraged as a public health measure (Addiction Research Foundation of Ontario and the Canadian Centre on Substance Abuse, 1994). Encouraging women to drink during pregnancy on this basis is unwarranted. The reader should consult the published literature for more information (Ashley et al., 1994; Fuchs et al., 1995; U.S. Department of Health and Human Services, 1993).

One of the basic techniques used in universal prevention is public education. Television advertisements, public service announcements, pamphlets, posters, and the like, which serve to educate the public about the risks of alcohol abuse and to encourage responsible drinking are universal prevention interventions that indirectly discourage use of alcohol during pregnancy. Universal prevention could also involve changes to the social environment (Single, 1987; Wallack, 1984), such as laws and regulations reinforcing norms and practices that depict heavy drinking and alcohol abuse as unacceptable.

The literature abuse indicates that higher socioeconomic status (SES), education, and access to meaningful employment are influential in decreasing the likelihood of alcohol abuse and, therefore, may lower FAS outcomes among women. Certainly *low SES is correlated* with FAS outcomes (Bingol et al., 1987; Sokol et al., 1980), ostensibly because the most highly abusive maternal drinking patterns are found among some individuals in low-SES groups. Although these problems may, in part, be generated by low SES, people who abuse alcohol might also drift to a lower SES. Consequently, universal prevention might be facilitated by improving social and economic opportunities for the entire population and reducing the prevalence of alcohol abuse. However, women of mid or high SES have given birth to children with FAS, ARBD, or ARND. No matter what the socioeconomic level, women who abuse alcohol are at risk for giving birth to an FAS baby.

The above examples are the types of prevention activities undertaken to decrease risk factors and increase protective factors for alcohol abuse in general; they are not specific to FAS. Given the high cost of alcohol-related problems in the United States—$85 billion in 1985, (U.S. Department of Health and Human Services, 1993)—these measures are valuable in and of themselves, apart from whatever impact they might have on FAS. Most certainly, these messages could influence the drinking behavior of some pregnant or preconceptional women.

Universal prevention of FAS further strives to ensure that all members of society understand that drinking during pregnancy can have hazardous consequences. Universal prevention promotes and supports positive, broadly shared attitudes and beliefs to protect the fetus from alcohol. Male partners and extended family members could play vital roles in the translation of these positive traits, as do peer groups (Wilsnack and Beckman, 1984; Wilsnack et al., 1991) and health care providers.

No universally safe level of alcohol consumption has been identified for pregnant women. Neither a specific level of alcohol consumption nor precise information on the biological, experiential, and behavioral characteristics of the mother of an FAS child has been well defined. At present, there is uncertainty whether minimal alcohol intake during pregnancy could be associated with any degree of injury to the baby. Some of the large research studies conducted in various cities in the United States have shown statistical associations between less than heavy levels of alcohol consumption by pregnant women and the birth and developmental outcomes in their offspring, the vast majority of whom have not been diagnosed with FAS, ARBD, or ARND (see Russell, 1991, for a review). For example, a study in Pittsburgh reports deficits in height and weight at age 3 associated statistically with moderate drinking (Day et al., 1991).

There are several issues relevant to the interpretation of these data related to relatively low levels of alcohol exposure and their translation into public health messages. First, statistical association is not proof of causality. That is, there are other factors associated with alcohol consumption during pregnancy that might be the cause of the abnormal outcome measures in the offspring. Some of the studies controlled for a variety of potential confounders, such as tobacco use, but not all of them did. As discussed in Chapter 1 it is not clear how clinically relevant some of the differences might be (Day et al., 1991; Russell, 1991). Finally, many of the more subtle differences in the child associated with low or moderate levels of alcohol intake during pregnancy are very common, and the association with alcohol exposure could be spurious. Assuming a causal relation with alcohol exposure could be erroneous. Although the effects of low levels of alcohol exposure during pregnancy are easier to study rigorously in one sense (the population of pregnant women who drink at low or moderate levels is much greater than the population who drinks very heavily), the subtle nature of some of the outcomes makes it difficult. The committee focused on conditions more closely associated with heavier levels of alcohol consumption. The reader is referred to the many excellent reviews of the effect of lower levels of prenatal exposure for further information (see for example, Jacobson and Jacobson, 1994; Russell, 1991).

Whether or not further research clarifies the relation between low to moderate levels of alcohol during pregnancy and adverse birth outcomes, the universal prevention message for FAS is a conservative one that encourages abstinence prior to conception and throughout pregnancy as the safest course. This was articulated by the Surgeon General in 1981 (U.S. Public Health Service, 1981). One can understand that the public health message encourages total abstinence. However, this message is potentially problematic for some individuals—women, their partners, and even some in the medical community—because it seems to contradict years of experience. Current data from three separate surveys suggest that approximately 20 percent of pregnant women drink alcohol at some level during pregnancy (CDC, 1995b; NIDA, 1994; Serdula et al., 1991). The vast majority of the babies born to these women show no overt signs of damage. Therefore, it is sometimes hard to convince these women that they should not have consumed alcohol or that they should not consume it during the next pregnancy.

Public health messages must be simple and can never fully explain the scientific and medical facts and uncertainties behind the message. If further research demonstrates a causal relation between low or moderate levels of alcohol consumption and less severe or complete manifestations of neurobehavioral damage than seen in FAS, ARBD, or ARND, as has been hypothesized, then this most conservative message of total abstinence will have been wise and reasonable.

An obvious example of a universal prevention intervention specific to FAS is warning labels on alcoholic beverages (see Box 7-1) or similar signs posted in restaurants or bars. These interventions are mandated by federal and state law. They are delivered to and accessible to everyone who drinks alcohol, including all pregnant women, not just those at high risk based on either population-based factors (selective prevention interventions) or individual factors (indicated prevention interventions) of delivering a baby with FAS. Many groups, such as the March of Dimes, the American College of Obstetrics and Gynecology, and drug store chains, have put out pamphlets with information about FAS; the National Organization on Fetal Alcohol Syndrome recently sponsored public service announcements about FAS by popular musicians Bonnie Raitt and Queen Latifah.

Health care providers can and should engage in universal prevention interventions. Visits to family practitioners and to obstetrician gynecologists offer the opportunity for brief messages about the importance of responsible alcohol use and for providing general information about the risks of alcohol to the fetus (American College of Obstetricians and Gynecologists, 1994). It should be stan-

---

BOX 7-1
Warning Label on Alcoholic Beverages

GOVERNMENT WARNING: (1) ACCORDING TO THE SURGEON GENERAL, WOMEN SHOULD NOT DRINK ALCOHOLIC BEVERAGES DURING PREGNANCY BECAUSE OF THE RISK OF BIRTH DEFECTS. (2) CONSUMPTION OF ALCOHOLIC BEVERAGES IMPAIRS YOUR ABILITY TO DRIVE A CAR OR OPERATE MACHINERY AND MAY CAUSE HEALTH PROBLEMS.

SOURCE: Public Law 100-690, Section 204.

---

dard medical practice to talk to women about their alcohol consumption (Cefalo and Moos, 1995; Mullen and Glenday, 1990) and this appears to be more common now than in the past. An increase in these activities is part of the Healthy People 2000 goals (see Table 1-1). As universal interventions such messages would be brief, delivered to every patient, and almost generic. More targeted messages and questioning would depend on whether the woman drinks and is pregnant. These are discussed under selective interventions.

While universal prevention activities in isolation may have had some effects, there has been no data found that demonstrates a change in the prevalence of FAS in response to such efforts. As discussed in Chapter 5, there are no definitive data on the prevalence or incidence of FAS. According to some surveys, its incidence appears to have increased (CDC, 1995a). This is most likely due to improvements in case identification, rather than a true increase in incidence. Therefore, as discussed in Chapter 5, proxy measures of the impact of prevention activities are appropriate to consider. Relevant proxy measures might include knowledge, attitudes, and beliefs, as well as prevalence of drinking by pregnant women.

Universal interventions seem to have increased the general knowledge of FAS and related problems. Data from the National Health Interview Survey indicate a statistically significant increase between 1985 and 1990 in the number of people ages 18 to 44 who had heard of FAS, who agreed that heavy drinking (as defined by each respondent) carries pregnancy-related risks, and who could correctly identify FAS as a birth defect (other choices were that the baby was born drunk or addicted to alcohol) (Dufour et al., 1994). However, those same data show that in 1990, a small percentage of people believe that FAS means that a baby is born drunk, 60 percent of all men and women between 18 and 44 years of age who had heard of FAS thought it referred to an alcohol-addicted baby, and only 29 percent of all women of childbearing age could correctly describe FAS as a birth defect.

Careful analysis of a study on the impact of the alcoholic beverage warning label on the drinking of approximately 3,500 pregnant women shows that after introduction of the warning label, pregnant women who drank very little (the equivalent of less than one mixed drink per day) decreased their alcohol consumption by an amount equivalent to 1 ounce of beer per week (Hankin, 1994). Pregnant women who drank more (the equivalent of more than one mixed drink per day) did not change their drinking behavior. These data suggest that universal prevention interventions might have little direct impact on FAS, ARBD, or ARND.

Data suggest that many women cut down their consumption of alcohol while pregnant (Serdula et al., 1991). Some pregnant women do not drink simply because the state of pregnancy decreases the palatability of alcohol for them. However, it is possible that increasing awareness of FAS and risks to the fetus have contributed to the decreases. Nevertheless, data indicate that women who drink heavily do not cut down their consumption of alcohol while pregnant. Because it is these women who are at risk for giving birth to an FAS child, it seems that universal prevention activities would have had little impact on the incidence of FAS. If future research suggests that low or modest levels of alcohol are associated with damage to the fetus other than FAS, ARBD, or ARND, then universal prevention interventions might decrease the incidence of those more subtle effects.

SELECTIVE PREVENTION INTERVENTIONS

Selective prevention interventions are targeted to people who are at greater risk for a particular outcome because they are members of a subgroup known to be at higher risk than the general population. These interventions involve different levels of targeting and intensity compared to universal prevention interventions. Some selective prevention is stimulated by general public information (universal prevention). A trickle-down effect of information may occur among those who are in a vulnerable state and thus at higher risk; and thus, the broadly dispersed universal prevention information on alcohol and pregnancy may or may not have a greater effect on vulnerable populations than on the general population. However, a trickle-down effect is not sufficient (Fitzgerald, 1988), and effective interventions must be devised to specifically target people who are members of high-risk groups.

Targets of selective prevention for FAS, ARBD, and ARND include women in the reproductive age range who drink alcohol. This is a very large and heterogeneous population. Chapter 6 includes a discussion on women's drinking and relevant risk factors. In general, a risk reduction approach to prevention and treatment of alcohol abuse in pregnancy would be strengthened by increased scientific knowledge about personal and social risk factors for drinking by pregnant women.

Population-Based Risk Factors for Giving Birth to an FAS Child

The epidemiologic literature related to FAS clearly identifies several risk factors for giving birth to an FAS child. First, and most obviously, is consumption while pregnant of large quantities of alcohol—either continuously or in risky patterns, such as bingeing–although there are many children diagnosed with FAS for whom a good history of maternal alcohol consumption is not available. For those women who have had a baby with FAS and for whom alcohol consumption is known, the levels, pattern, and frequency of alcohol consumed have typically been high. However, as described in Chapter 5, a high proportion of women who abuse alcohol while pregnant do not give birth to a child with FAS. Alcohol is not unlike most teratogens in that not all fetuses, not even dizygotic twins, are equally affected by the same amount of exposure. The epidemiologic literature identifies other risk factors for alcohol use during pregnancy: age, race, marital status, smoking level, and SES (see Chapter 6). Special selective prevention interventions could be designed based on these factors.

Role of the Father

Because the Committee to Study Fetal Alcohol Syndrome views the targets of FAS prevention activities as appropriately including more than just women, the partners of women who drink could be included in selective prevention activities as well. In contrast to the attention devoted to the influence of maternal factors on pregnancy outcome, data on the possible role of paternal factors are sparse. The association between alcohol exposure in utero and FAS, ARBD, and ARND is well established. Maternal alcohol exposure causes FAS. Similarly, the important social, psychological, and behaviorally supportive role that the male partner plays in a healthy pregnancy is well established and cannot be emphasized too strongly. However, the possible biophysiological contribution of paternal alcohol consumption to an adverse pregnancy outcome is not well understood. The animal literature suggests that male exposure to alcohol might result in some damage to sperm, and thus affect the fetus. Data from animal models suggest that paternal alcohol exposure may affect organ weights, hormone secretion, and immune response in the offspring (Abel, 1993; Abel and Blitzke, 1990; Abel and Tan, 1986; Cicero, 1994; Hazlett et al., 1989), but paternal consumption of alcohol does not cause FAS.

Since women who drink heavily tend to associate with men who also drink heavily (Jacob and Premer, 1986; Russell, 1991), and many children with FAS have fathers who abuse alcohol (Abel, 1983), there is a possibility that some of the anomalies now attributed to the teratogenic effects of maternal drinking may be exacerbated by paternal drinking. Clarification of this issue, including the possible mechanisms of paternal alcohol effects, awaits further research.

Regardless of whether future research indicates a direct role for prenatal paternal alcohol exposure in birth defects other than FAS, ARBD, and ARND, prevention efforts directed at men are appropriate and important for the influences that men have on women's drinking. For men, emphasis could be placed on the important social, psychological, and behavioral role they can play in supporting a healthy pregnancy. When appropriate, men should be encouraged to enter treatment for alcohol abuse, both for their own health and well-being and to make it easier for the pregnant woman to stop drinking. However, since many women who are at high risk for FAS are unmarried, in very unstable relationships, or both, it is important to tailor interventions to these situations. Contracts with other significant persons or with an entire at-risk community might be useful, including extended family, influential peers, and possibly bartenders. Boxes 7-2 and 7-3 represent family- and community-wide pledges related to drinking during pregnancy that are used by two Native American communities. These approaches seem to have promise for some communities but have not been evaluated.

BOX 7-2
Sample Vision and Mission Statements

Here is an excellent example of a vision and mission statement developed by the prevention leaders of the American Indian reservation community of Zuni Pueblo, New Mexico. It is positive, uplifting, value-oriented, and it encapsulates the cultural and humanitarian reasons for their FAS prevention efforts. It is also accompanied by a four-page list of problem statements, goals, objectives, barriers to overcome, and outcome measures.

Vision Statement

Zuni will be a community that affirms and accepts the cultural values of the sanctity of life and the values of women's and men's roles in nurturing the healthy development of infants and children. Young people will promote supportive roles for each other in developing healthy lifestyles with a sense of unity within the community.

Mission Statement

"Keep the tradition by working together for generations of healthy babies." The FAS Coalition will promote the coordination of community services for prenatals and their families. Community resources will be committed to helping young people create healthy lifestyles within the Zuni culture.

(Pueblo of Zuni, 1993)

BOX 7-3
Family Pledge: Spokane Tribal Fetal Alcohol Syndrome/
Fetal Alcohol Effect Office

- MY FAMILY IS THE MOST IMPORTANT PART OF MY LIFE.
- MY FAMILY INCLUDES ALL THOSE BORN BEFORE ME,
  ALL THOSE BORN SINCE MY AND BIRTH AND
  ALL THOSE THAT HAVE YET TO BE BORN.
- I WILL DO ALL I CAN TO PROTECT MY FAMILY FROM HARM.
- I WILL PROTECT THOSE YET TO BE BORN BY BEHAVING AS
  A WARRIOR.
- TRADITIONAL INDIAN BELIEF HOLDS THAT ALL WOMEN AND
  CHILDREN ARE SACRED AND RESPONSIBLE FOR THE FAMILY'S
  ANCESTRAL SURVIVAL.
- AS A WARRIOR, I WILL PROTECT THE UNBORN CHILD FROM THE
  EFFECTS OF ALCOHOL BY NOT DRINKING ALCOHOL MYSELF OR
  SEEING THAT THOSE WITH CHILD DO NOT DRINK ALCOHOL.
- BY SIGNING THIS, I SWEAR ON MY FAMILY'S HONOR TO KEEP THIS
  PLEDGE.

SIGNED _____   DATE _____

SOURCE: Fetal Alcohol Prevention and Education Family Album, Developed by
the Spokane Tribe of Indians Fetal Alcohol Program; Spokane Tribal Community
Action Team, Wellpinit, Washington.

Role of Health Care Professionals

Finally, increasing the awareness of health care providers will indirectly act as prevention interventions. Health care providers should be encouraged and educated about FAS. Clinicians should be trained to question women in an appropriate manner about their drinking and contraceptive histories. If a woman drinks alcohol and has other risk factors for FAS, health care providers should deliver selective or indicated prevention interventions, and this requires training and preparation. Clinicians should be prepared not just to question women about their alcohol abuse, but to discuss all aspects of alcohol use. This could serve to advise women who deny an alcohol abuse problem and to reassure those who might have had very minimal exposure before pregnancy was recognized. This might alleviate guilt in some women who don't understand the magnitude of exposure associated with fetal risk.

While it is easiest to identify alcohol-related problems among those who are most severely affected, the challenge for primary health care providers is to identify affected individuals early in their involvement and to intervene in a timely and meaningful manner. The importance of screening for problem use of alcohol and the role of the primary health care professional in prevention, brief office interventions, and referrals for formal treatment cannot be overemphasized.

The primary health care provider can play an important role in the identification of alcohol-related problems in women. Obstetrician gynecologists and other primary health practitioners who provide health care to women often serve as counselors for questions and concerns related to women's general health and reproduction, and have opportunities to advise women about the potential risks of alcohol use. Annual routine health visits and pre- and postnatal visits provide multiple opportunities to discuss alcohol and the effects of alcohol consumption on health. Routine questions about and assessment of alcohol intake give women opportunities to ask questions about drinking during pregnancy and provide health care providers with opportunities to give advice and address the health of women whose alcohol use may put them at risk for adverse outcomes, especially during pregnancy. Such questioning is recommended as standard procedure in preconceptional and prenatal care.

Screening Instruments

The purpose of screening is to identify health problems or risks in time for intervention to prevent serious consequences such as FAS. Several screening tools are available to help identify women who potentially have alcohol abuse problems. Someone who is likely to be an alcohol abuser as indicated by screening should undergo a more thorough assessment of her alcohol use. Relevant information would include, for example, quantity, frequency, and pattern of alcohol use, and level of dependence.

Several authors recommend the use of the CAGE test (see Box 7-4). The

---

BOX 7-4
***CAGE* Test**

C Have you ever felt you ought to *Cut Down* on your drinking?
A Have people ever *Annoyed* you by criticizing your drinking?
G Have you ever felt bad or *Guilty* about your drinking?
E Have you ever had a drink first thing in the morning to steady your nerves or get rid of a hangover (*Eye-Opener*)?

The *CAGE* test is a screening tool for identifying risk drinkers. Each positive answer is scored as 1 point. 2 or more points is considered as evidence of possible risk drinking.

SOURCE: Ewing JA. Detecting alcoholism: The CAGE questionnaire. Journal of the American Medical Association 1984:252;1905-1907.

BOX 7-5
T-ACE Test

T How many drinks does it take to make you feel high (*Tolerance*)?
A Have people ever *Annoyed* you by criticizing your drinking?
C Have you ever felt you ought to *Cut Down* on your drinking?
E Have you ever had a drink first thing in the morning to steady your nerves or get rid of a hangover (*Eye-Opener*)?

The *T-ACE* test is a screening tool for identifying risk drinkers. The Tolerance question is scored as 2 points if the respondent reports needing more than two drinks to get high. The other questions are scored as 1 point each for a positive answer. Scores of 2 or more are considered evidence of risk drinking.

SOURCE: Sokol RJ, Martier SS, Ager JW. The T-ACE questions: practical prenatal detection of risk-drinking. American Journal of Obstetrics and Gynecology 1989;160:863-868; discussion, pp. 868-870.

BOX 7-6
TWEAK Test

T *Tolerance:* How many drinks can you hold?
W Have close friends or relatives *Worried* or complained about your drinking in the past year?
E *Eye-Opener:* Do you sometimes take a drink in the morning when you first get up?
A *Amnesia:* Has a friend or family member ever told you about things you said or did while you were drinking that you could not remember?
K(C) Do you sometimes feel the need to *Cut Down* on your drinking?

A 7-point scale is used to score the test. The Tolerance question scores 2 points if the responding reports the ability to hold more than five drinks without falling asleep or passing out. A positive response to the Worry question scores 2 points, and a positive response to the last three questions scores 1 point each. A total of 2 or more points indicates the respondent is likely to be a risk drinker.

SOURCE: Russell M. New assessment tools for risk drinking during pregnancy. Alcohol Health and Research World 1994; 18:55-61.

CAGE is an easily remembered mnemonic representing four brief questions that can be incorporated into routine practice (Ewing, 1984). The CAGE questions have proven useful in screening for alcoholism. The questions focus on **cutting down** on drinking, **annoyance** at criticism by others about drinking, **guilty** feelings about drinking or something done while drinking, and the use of an **eye-opener**. Although a positive response to the CAGE questions is not diagnostic of alcohol use disorders, answering yes to two or more questions is highly suspicious and warrants further evaluation. These steps are discussed under indicated prevention.

Another common screening test for alcoholism in adults is the Michigan Alcoholism Screening Test (MAST), a series of 25 questions, many drawn from earlier alcoholism surveys (Selzer, 1971). Alcohol screening tests such as the MAST and the CAGE, although not designed to screen pregnant women, have served as sources of items for other questionnaires that have been found useful in screening for at-risk drinking during pregnancy.

A variant of the CAGE, referred to as the T-ACE (see Box 7-5) substitutes **tolerance** for the question on guilt (How many drinks does it take to make you feel high?). The sensitivity of this simple four question screening test in gravid women who admitted to having had a drink of alcohol was such that it was able to detect 7 out of 10 women who drank enough to constitute an embryonic fetal risk. Another brief screening test, the TWEAK, has been found to be somewhat more sensitive but less specific in identifying women who are risk drinkers (Russell, 1994; see Box 7-6). It combines questions from the MAST, CAGE, and T-ACE tests that have been found to be most effective in identifying high-risk women drinkers (Russell, 1994).

Biomarkers

Given the limits of self-reports of alcohol use in many circumstances, an efficient, nonintrusive, valid, and inexpensive biologic marker of alcohol use would be an important tool for alcohol treatment research. Moreover, the availability of biomarkers might lead to earlier interventions for preventing FAS, serve as an indicator for evaluating FAS prevention outcomes, help identify instances of maternal under-reporting of alcohol use, and facilitate research on possible dose-response relations between alcohol exposure and adverse health effects, including FAS, ARBD, and ARND.

Although research continues to search for an ideal biomarker of alcohol exposure, no satisfactory laboratory test currently exists. Other issues concerning the applicability of biomarkers to women who drink during pregnancy, for example how to reach many of the women who give birth to FAS infants, need to be considered. Furthermore, suggesting such screening may pose difficulties for the relationship between the physician and the pregnant woman making further prenatal care less likely. This is vitally important given their lack of prenatal care and usual entrance into the health care system at a late stage of pregnancy. A biomarker for alcohol abuse would not be a substitute for a health care provider's verbal assessment of alcohol use by at-risk women. Such interaction can sometimes be the first step in developing a supportive relationship that could be crucial to the woman's progress in achieving abstinence or, at least, moderation. Biomarkers can be very useful for research purposes. For example, they could help establish dose-response relations for prenatal alcohol exposure and adverse fetal outcome and could help delineate effects of alcohol from other confounders.

Studies will need to continue to explore the validity and efficiency of possible tests, examine the specific impact of pregnancy in addition to gender, as well as the impact of other confounding variables including nutrition, age, parity, smoking, other substance abuse, and preexisting illnesses and conditions. The validity of biomarkers is based on both a test's degree of sensitivity and specificity of an exposure. Sensitivity represents a test's ability to identify correctly those who have been exposed or who have the disease, while the specificity of a test identifies correctly those who have not been exposed or who do not have the disease (Mausner and Kramer, 1985).

To date, several laboratory tests, including blood alcohol levels, creatine phosphokinase, D-glucaric acid, urinary dolichol, and erythrocyte δ-aminolevulinic acid dehydrase, are being explored as possible markers. Some may indicate recent alcohol exposure, other chronic alcohol exposure, and other liver damage, the latter finding suggesting possible chronic alcohol abuse. Overall, however, the clinical usefulness of these markers thus far have been less than promising.

The breath analyzer measures alcohol in the breath and has become the "gold standard" for detecting recent consumption of alcohol. However, blood alcohol levels are only reliable when blood is tested within the first 24 hours of the ingestion and are of limited value in diagnosing chronic alcohol abuse. Creatine phosphokinase (CPK) is an enzyme found in large quantities in the brain and in skeletal and cardiac muscle, but is absent from the liver. Fifty percent of all alcoholics appear to have elevated levels of CPK. Unlike many markers, therefore, CPK can be elevated with or without liver disease since it is not an index of liver function. However, due to confounding variables among alcoholics, CPK is considered both insensitive and nonspecific for diagnosing chronic alcohol abuse and alcoholism. D-Glucaric acid is the end product of glucuronic acid metabolism. When alcohol is ingested, the alcohol becomes a catalyst inducing the enzymes involved in the synthesis of D-glucaric acid allowing urinary D-glucaric acid levels to be used as screening tests for alcohol abuse. Unfortunately, discrepancies have been reported which would limit the validity of this test (Mihas and Tavassoli, 1992).

Urinary dolichol and erythrocyte δ-aminolevulinic acid dehydrase tests are still under investigation as possible biomarkers for alcohol exposure. Although urinary dolichol has been found to be an indicator of alcohol abuse among chronic alcoholics and in their offspring, dolichol levels can be confounded by age, Alzheimer's disease, and metastatic cancers, thus decreasing the sensitivity and specificity of the test. Erythrocyte δ-aminolevulinic (ALA) acid dehydrase is an enzyme involved in heme biosynthesis that has been found to be lowered in over 90% of alcoholics. Erythrocyte ALA dehydrase activity does remain depressed for approximately 1 week in alcoholics after withdrawal from alcohol but only for 24 hours in nonalcoholics. As a result, laborious (and therefore expensive) methodology and the time-dependent nature of the test have hampered its use in clinical settings as an appropriate test for alcohol abuse (Mihas and Tavassoli, 1992).

Several promising markers for detecting alcohol consumption and abuse include gamma glutamyl transferase (GGT), aspartate aminotransferase (AST), alanine aminotransferase (ALT), alkaline phosphatase (AP), mean corpuscular volume (MCV), acetaldehyde adducts, and carbohydrate-deficient transferrin (CDT). These are described in more detail here. Studies indicate that several of these tests, particularly in combination, show sensitivity and specificity. Several have been analyzed for gender differences and the effect of pregnancy and one has been analyzed for its relation to fetal outcome.

Gamma glutamyl transferase   GGT is a cell-membrane bound glycoprotein that catalyzes the transfer of the gamma-glutamyl moiety of glutathione to the various peptide acceptors. GGT is found in various tissues throughout the body including the liver, kidney, spleen, pancreas, brain, and heart (Mihas and Tavassoli, 1992). Although the mechanism by which serum GGT is heightened from chronic alcohol consumption has yet to be defined, GGT has become a widely used laboratory screening test for alcohol abuse and alcoholism because of its proven sensitivity (39-78%) and specificity (11-50%) in detecting alcoholic liver disease (Gjerde et al., 1988; Stibler et al., 1979). However, the validity of the test may be hampered by the fact that elevated GGT serum levels occur in both alcoholic and nonalcoholic liver disease, as well as in individuals taking drugs that induce hepatic enzymes (Mihas and Tavassoli, 1992).

Aminotransferases   Aspartate aminotransferase (AST) or glutamate oxaloacetate transaminase and its correlate, alanine aminotransferase (ALT), represent the most frequently measured enzymes for liver disease and the most sensitive indicators of hepatocyte necrosis. Serum AST becomes elevated as result of abnormal hepatocellular membrane permeability and leakage and has been found in patients with all forms of liver disease. However, since toxic effects of alcohol may also manifest itself in other organs besides the liver, the incidence of elevated serum AST varies significantly among alcoholics and has a sensitivity value of 31-64%, as well as an extremely low specificity since it will be elevated with liver disease of any kind. As a result, AST is viewed as an unreliable marker when used alone. Mitochondrial AST has, however, proven to be effective in recognizing alcoholic liver disease because the mitochondrial toxicity of alcohol occurs before liver cell necrosis takes place (Mihas and Tavassoli, 1992). On the other hand, the mitochondrial correlate of ALT, alanine aminotransferase, however, has not proven to be a useful marker of chronic alcoholism or of alcoholic liver disease with a sensitivity range of 37-47% and low specificity (Gjerde et al., 1988; Stibler et al., 1979). In theory, the ratio of ALT to AST may be of some use.

Alkaline Phosphatase Alkaline phosphatase (AP) is an enzyme that hydrolyzes organic phosphate esters in an alkaline environment creating an organic radical and inorganic phosphate. Present in most organs of the body, AP's elevation in liver disease due primarily to cholestatic disorders does not allow for distinction between intrahepatic and extrahepatic sources. The ratio of AP to GGT has been used as a rather sensitive marker of excessive consumption of alcohol, but the incomplete understanding of its biosynthesis has limited its value in diagnosing patients (Mihas and Tavassoli, 1992).

Mean Corpuscular Volume Many alcoholic patients have an elevated erythrocyte mean corpuscular volume (MCV) and mean red cell hemoglobin, as well as the presence of macrocytosis. The elevations are attributed to the direct effect of alcohol on developing erythroblasts and indirectly to the presence of folate deficiency. Simultaneously, macrocytosis will occur and persist until all alcohol consumption has stopped. Alone, the sensitivity of MCV is 26-71% and the specificity is 20-74% and has been found to detect only 30-40% of subjects with an alcohol problem. However, MCV, combined with other laboratory tests such as GGT and AP, appears to improve one's ability to detect chronic alcohol abusers (Harouki et al., 1983; Stibler et al., 1979).

Acetaldehyde adducts Acetaldehyde adducts form in the liver during chronic exposure to alcohol due to the activity of ethanol dehydrogenase and a microsomal ethanol oxidizing system. Currently, further tests are needed to assess the validity and usefulness of acetaldehyde adducts as a marker of chronic alcohol abuse and alcoholism. Blood acetate levels examine the byproduct, acetate, of alcohol oxidation which does not become metabolized in the liver. As the body attempts to eliminate alcohol from its system, a metabolic tolerance to alcohol occurs in the blood (Mihas and Tavassoli, 1992). The acetaldehyde adducts are measured usually in whole blood (WBAA) or as hemoglobin adducts (HbAA). With a sensitivity of 65% and a specificity of 92%, the test surpasses gamma glutamyl transferase (GGT) values making the blood acetate levels one of the leading biomarkers to detect early alcoholism (Korri et al., 1985).

A recent study demonstrated significant differences in WBAA levels between the general population and people who don't drink and between the general population and subjects enrolled in an outpatient alcohol treatment program

(Halvorsen et al., 1993a). Another study compared HbAA levels with results from the Self-Administered Alcoholism Screening Test (SAAST) in people who were abstinent, self-defined social drinkers, and people reporting for treatment for alcoholism (Peterson et al., 1990). Both analyses could distinguish the alcoholic group from the abstinent group and from the social drinkers. There was no difference between the abstinent group and the social drinkers. Although both measures correlated with each other, the SAAST seemed to be the more sensitive test.

Males have higher WBAA levels than women (Halvorsen et al., 1993b) and this gender difference is seen in the general population and in populations that don't drink (Halvorsen et al., 1993a). HbAA levels also increase with age, and this correlation is stronger for women than men.

HbAA levels have been studied in pregnant women who were followed until delivery (Niemala et al., 1991). The offspring were assessed and of 19 alcohol abusing women, 8 had infants diagnosed as having "fetal alcohol effects." HbAA levels were elevated in 68 percent of women who had alcohol-affected babies but only in 28 percent of the mothers who abused alcohol while pregnant but gave birth to non-affected babies.

Carbohydrate-deficient Transferrin   Transferrin acts as the major iron transport of protein in the biological fluids of all vertebrates. Reduced contents of sialic acid cause an increase in the amount of higher isoelectric points than normal. These characteristics are readily detectable through separation by charge. Carbohydrate-deficient transferrin (CDT) for example is deficient in the terminal trisaccharide and can be distinguished its from transferrin by isoelectric point (Mihas and Tavassoli, 1992).

During subacute heavy alcohol consumption, CDT, a deglycosylated form of the liver synthesized protein transferrin, is produced and can be detected using conventional anion exchanger and radioimmunoassay technology. CDT levels do not return to normal for 2 to 3 weeks and thus is a marker of present or recent alcohol abuse, and occurs irrespective of liver disease. Following extensive testing and comparison with other biomarkers, CDT has proved to be one of the most sensitive and specific markers for chronic alcoholism with values ranging from 83-90% and 99-100% respectively (Stibler et al., 1979; Storey et al., 1987). It has been found that consumption of as little as 20 g/day of alcohol can be detected through CDT (Mihas and Tavassoli, 1992). These studies have indicated that this marker may be a more sensitive and specific indicator of alcohol abuse than the more established GGT (Anton and Moak, 1994).

In many studies, CDT has been described as being more specific and sensitive than GGT. However, both CDT and GGT have been found to discriminate between the sexes indicating a lower specificity in women for both tests. For years, studies have shown that GGT is normally lower in females than males, and that an elevated GGT level correlated with an increase in alcohol consumption, but at greater levels in men compared to women. CDT was also found to have a lower sensitivity among women than in men (Anton and Moak, 1994).

It is imperative to understand the gender differences for these tests as more and more women present for and enter treatment. The seriousness of the consequences from alcohol abuse by women directly impacts their own health, as well as the health of their fetuses, during pregnancy. As a result, several studies, including one by Anton and Moak (1994), indicated that when GGT is combined with CDT, the sensitivity for detecting heavy alcohol consumption is improved among women, without losing specificity. Studies have also examined the possibility of confounding variables among women including the use of oral contraceptives and being pregnant or of menopausal status. Examining only CDT levels, these studies did not reveal that the above variables significantly influence CDT levels. However, it has been suggested that pregnancy decreases CDT, an effect opposite to alcohol consumption. Related studies, however, indicate that intake of estrogen or progesterone is likely to increase CDT levels and bias the results. Iron deficiency anemia, a quite prevalent condition in many women secondary to menstrual loss and pregnancy, may increase the total transferrin present (Anton and Moak, 1994). However, further studies are needed to explore this relationship and the impact of detecting alcohol abuse among women and especially among pregnant women. Without thorough investigation of the impact of pregnancy upon these tests it is impossible to make specific recommendations at this time for use in prenatal clinic.

Brief Interventions and Referral

Assessing risk during pregnancy through screening is an essential step toward educating pregnant women about the potential dangers of such behaviors. Once a problem has been identified, the health provider must make an appropriate intervention or treatment referral. Options range from brief interventions offered during the office visit to referral to a treatment specialist or a treatment program. The strength of the intervention should be proportional to the risk. In a stepped-care approach, intervention begins with the least intensive level of treatment for all affected individuals (e.g., brief interventions), with the provision of increasingly intensive levels of intervention (e.g., day treatment or hospitalization) for those who do not respond to lower treatment levels or who show evidence of alcohol dependence.

Justification to support the utility of health guidance and early intervention to prevent or treat alcohol abuse, comes from the belief that health messages provided by physicians, as sources of credible information, can affect behavioral change in alcohol use. Health messages offered by primary health care providers reinforce information already received from mass media or other group settings. Reinforcement of these messages in various settings has a greater effect on behavioral change than do prevention interventions delivered by only one source. Lessons learned from smoking cessation intervention are a good example of this.

Effective brief interventions typically include an initial evaluation after which the patient is given structured feedback about her situation. This provides the patient with the opportunity to reflect in detail upon her present situation. Brief interventions also emphasize the patient's responsibility for change. A third common element is giving clear advice to the patient to make a change with a specific goal such as total abstinence, elimination of hazardous use, or seeking treatment. Alternatively, the patient can be presented with a menu of alternative strategies for changing alcohol or other drug use. Although providing advice is important, the patient must ultimately make the decision to change her alcohol use. Effective brief interventions also typically emphasize the empathic nature of the health care provider-patient relationships and seek to reinforce the patient's self-efficacy or optimism.

Interventions for alcohol problems should provide a patient with the necessary information, skills, and support to help her overcome barriers and utilize resources in order to change her behavior. Overtly directive and confrontational styles tend to evoke high levels of patient resistance, whereas a more empathic style is associated with less resistance and better long-term change (Miller and Rollnick, 1991).

The incorporation of simple screening tests and, where appropriate, brief interventions and referral for treatment, into the routine history taking of patients is advocated for all primary health care providers and can help in early identification of women with potential drinking problems. Brief interventions or referral to professionals trained in assessing and treating women who abuse alcohol may be the first steps toward recovery for some patients.

Professional Education

Although routine screening for alcohol use may be a desirable goal, much will have to change before it becomes a reality. Numerous studies show that physicians are uncomfortable with, and report a need for additional training in screening and management of alcohol-related problems. Educational programs should help primary care practitioners develop the clinical skills to assess and manage patients with alcohol problems. At a minimum, curricular time should be devoted to alcohol-related issues in medical schools, residency training programs, and continuing medical education courses (Adger et al., 1990).

Physicians and other health professionals in training need to develop a sense of responsibility and optimism toward their patients' alcohol or other substance abuse and confidence in their clinical skills related to caring for patients with these problems. Practitioners will develop these qualities only if they have adequate clinical exposure to patients who abuse alcohol (Bradley and Larson, 1994).

An FAS curriculum developed by the National Organization on Fetal Alcohol Syndrome (NOFAS) and the Center on Alcoholism, Substance Abuse, and Addictions at the University of New Mexico was pilot tested at the university's medical school in Albuquerque in 1992, and an adapted version has been in use there ever since. In addition, Georgetown University Medical School has offered the course for two years, and Northwestern University Medical School began offering it in 1995. The class includes both lecture and clinical activities. The goal is to provide a core knowledge of FAS, to teach recognition of FAS, and to improve skills both in detecting pregnant women's use of alcohol or other drugs and in counseling women about such use. Students are tested for relevant knowledge before and after the unit. Each school tailors the course to its own curriculum. The Northwestern program, for example, has been adapted in keeping with its problem-based learning approach. NOFAS hopes to extend use of the curriculum to additional medical schools as well as to nursing schools and nurse-midwife programs.

The national Residency Review Committee for Obstetrics and Gynecology now requires that residency programs include instruction on behavioral medicine and psychosocial problems, including substance abuse. The March of Dimes Birth Defects Foundation has produced a curriculum on substance abuse in pregnancy for use in such residency programs. It was developed in 1991 by the Greater New York March of Dimes and has been tested at a number of medical schools in New York City. The program is intended to improve the identification, care, and treatment of chemically dependent pregnant women and their children. It includes units on diagnosis of alcohol or other substance abuse, intervention and referral for such abuse, and relevant legal and ethical issues. The March of Dimes plans to publish the material and circulate it to residency programs in obstetrics and gynecology throughout the country.

Empirical Evaluation

There are studies showing that women who drink moderately or heavily are amenable to interventions offered in conjunction with prenatal care. Researchers at the Boston City Hospital Prenatal Clinic showed that counseling about drinking during pregnancy at routine prenatal visits led to decreases in alcohol use during pregnancy (Rosett et al., 1981a,b). The program offered counseling to women who were classified as heavy drinkers (5 or 6 drinks on some occasions and at least 45 drinks per month) and was oriented toward positive messages—stressing the increased likelihood of a healthy baby if the woman quit or decreased drinking, and improving the woman's self-esteem. Of 39 women who were counseled 3 or more times, over half were able to abstain or significantly moderate consumption of alcohol before the third trimester. Far fewer of the offspring born to the women who abstained or moderated their alcohol exposure were at or below the tenth percentile for growth measures than infants born to women who continued to drink heavily throughout pregnancy. This program was seminal in showing that pregnant women who abuse alcohol could successfully be counseled to reduce their abuse and improve infant outcome.

In a research project at Grady Memorial Hospital in Atlanta, women who applied for prenatal care during a 33-month period in the early 1980s were asked about alcohol use (Smith et al., 1987). Most of these women were in their second trimester. All women were counseled about the negative effects of alcohol, tobacco, and other drug use on their infants and were advised to stop using these substances. Women troubled by the information or identified as having significant substance abuse problems were referred for supportive counseling. One-third of the women who received intervention stopped drinking for the duration of their pregnancy. Compared with those who stopped drinking, women who drank throughout pregnancy reported having started drinking at a younger age, were more likely to report heavy drinking on the part of their parents and siblings (especially their female relatives), had more evidence of alcohol-related physical problems, and were more likely to qualify for a diagnosis of alcohol dependence based on the third edition of the Diagnostic and Statistical Manual (DSM-III) (American Psychiatric Association [APA], 1980). These data and others suggest that interventions during pregnancy can lead some women to stop drinking. However, there are no clear data to predict who will respond to such interventions and who will continue to drink. Such information could be useful in targeting interventions.

A pregnant woman who scores positive on a brief screening and has other risk factors should be educated about FAS. This education should be more specific or more involved than that delivered routinely to every pregnant woman. Following a more detailed assessment of risk, interventions should be planned. These interventions will range, as appropriate, from brief interventions to intensive inpatient treatment for alcohol dependence. Epidemiologic literature shows that most women cut down on their drinking during pregnancy (CDC, 1995b). Whether this is secondary to a brief intervention by a health care provider is not known. Pregnancy is known to be an opportune time for many health interventions—women are more open to changes in their lives to help increase the likelihood of a healthy pregnancy (Cefalo and Moos, 1995; IOM, 1995; Mullen and Glenday, 1990).

Whether such interventions would decrease the incidence of FAS, ARBD, or ARND is not clear, since women who drink only moderately and who easily quit or cut down might not be those who would have gone on to have an FAS child, because their consumption levels or patterns are not sufficient to cause FAS. It is difficult to test this in controlled studies because the number of women needed in a study to identify a change in FAS rate would be quite large, and such a study would be very expensive. Whether decreasing consumption in moderate drinkers would decrease problems is not clear; some studies show better birth outcomes in women who stopped drinking during pregnancy compared with those who drank heavily throughout pregnancy (Smith et al., 1987). Infants of women who continued to drink had a higher frequency of intrauterine growth retardation and neurobehavioral and morphological alterations (Coles et al., 1985, 1987; Smith et al., 1986). Many showed evidence of neonatal withdrawal syndrome as well (Coles et al., 1984). Follow-up showed a greater prevalence of developmental delays for those children whose mothers continued to drink throughout pregnancy (Brown et al., 1991; Coles et al., 1991).

INDICATED PREVENTION INTERVENTIONS

Indicated prevention interventions are targeted to high-risk individuals who are identified as having minimal but detectable signs or symptoms foreshadowing a condition or who have biological markers indicating predisposition (IOM, 1994). Studies show that a small proportion of women within some communities give birth to most of the FAS children (May et al., 1983). At present, the only biologic marker to identify an individual woman at high risk for giving birth to an FAS baby is having already given birth to an FAS child (May, in press). There is no prenatal test of fetal damage from alcohol that could be used to indicate a mother who should be aggressively treated to prevent further damage to the child.

The committee therefore considers the target for indicated prevention interventions to be a woman who abuses alcohol, including engaging in occasional binge drinking, while pregnant or at risk for being pregnant, particularly a pregnant or preconceptional woman who drinks alcohol and has already given birth to a child with FAS, ARBD, or ARND. As with selective interventions, the committee would also include interventions aimed at the partner, significant friends, or family members of a woman who fits the profile just described. Although other frameworks for describing prevention activities draw a line between prevention activities and treatment, indicated *prevention* of FAS includes *treatment* for alcohol abuse in a pregnant woman or for a woman highly likely to become pregnant. Thus, discussions about alcohol treatment for pregnant women and treatment outcome research are included in this chapter on prevention.

A first step in these prevention interventions is to identify the target. Brief screening tools for identifying high-risk women drinkers were described in the previous section. Women who score positive on such a screening tool should be given further assessment and consideration of a range of interventions ranging from brief interventions to formal treatment to encourage them to stop drinking. In cases where alcohol dependence, as described in DSM-IV, is diagnosed, referral for formal treatment should be made immediately. If brief interventions are indicated and on follow-up the woman continues to abuse alcohol, more intensive and targeted interventions including referral for formal alcohol abuse treatment should be called into play immediately. Women who abuse alcohol during pregnancy provide special challenges and thus far have been immune to most efforts to get them to stop or significantly reduce their drinking on their own. The committee identified little controlled research into the most effective ways to treat pregnant women who abuse alcohol.

Indicated prevention can also be promoted through intensive professional education (Bowen and Sammons, 1988; Davis and Frost, 1984; Little et al., 1981). Recognition by professionals engaged in human services of maternal drinking and of risky practices might be effective in FAS prevention efforts. It is important to educate professionals in addition to obstetrician gynecologists, because many women who have FAS babies have woefully inadequate or nonexistent prenatal care and often do not seek obstetric services until delivery. Therefore, any health care provider who comes in contact with women who abuse alcohol should consider brief intervention therapies and referral to more formal alcohol abuse treatment, if appropriate, and counsel her regarding the risks of prenatal alcohol exposure. Women of reproductive age who abuse alcohol should also be offered referral and access to birth control information and services. Since prenatal alcohol damage involves two major behaviors, conception and alcohol consumption, separating the two behaviors is preventive for FAS (Masis and May, 1991). All forms of birth control, from short term to permanent, need to be offered and available to at-risk females and partners alike. In recent years, some FAS prevention projects of the Centers for Disease Control and Prevention (CDC) include contraception as part of the package of prevention services being studied. There are no data, yet, to show whether education and availability of contraception as part of a comprehensive FAS prevention program will decrease FAS, ARBD, or ARND.

Women Who Have Given Birth to a Child with FAS, ARBD, or ARND

The type and intensity of a preventive intervention should be appropriate to the risk involved; thus, intensive actions should be considered for a woman who has given birth to a diagnosed FAS child. In these cases, because of possible stigmatization of the mother or the child, as discussed in other sections of this report, diagnoses should be assigned conservatively by qualified dysmorphologists or other clinicians skilled in the diagnosis of FAS. Diagnostic criteria put forth in this report should be used for assessment purposes. However, once a verified case of FAS has been identified, intensive measures must be taken to reduce the impairment and disability that might accumulate with successive pregnancies and constitute a heavy burden on society and on the woman's health and well-being.

FAS studies consistently report that women who have had one definite FAS child, and who continue to drink, have progressively more severely affected children with subsequent pregnancies (Abel, 1988; Davis and Lipson, 1984; May et al., 1983). Subsequent pregnancies with similar levels of alcohol consumption generally produce more severely affected children, because both parity and age contribute to the extent of damage (Abel and Sokol, 1986; May et al., 1983). The contribution of age might, in part, be related to length of time of alcohol abuse and the consequent liver damage. Intervention is best accomplished by assisting the mother (and, if possible, her partner) to change her substance use patterns, childbearing behavior, or both.

Some new research in this area might shed light on how best to do this. There are currently at least two controlled research projects comparing intensive versus standard education interventions. The project at Wayne State University includes women who had given birth to a child who did not necessarily have FAS, but who had admitted to drinking at high risk levels during that pregnancy; another, at University of Washington, involves women who have given birth to a child with FAS. These projects are new, and no results are available yet. However, it is not clear that the women in the first project are those who would give birth to an FAS baby and that widespread use of this type of intervention strategy would decrease FAS. If further research indicates more definitively prenatal effects of alcohol exposure at levels less than that which causes FAS, ARBD, or ARND, then decreases in drinking of any sort would be a valuable goal of prevention intervention for birth defects.

There have been some attempts at forced treatment and incarceration of pregnant woman who abuse illegal substances, particularly crack cocaine. These measures raise complicated ethical and legal questions. Mandated incarceration might decrease exposure of a particular fetus to alcohol (although alcohol and other drugs frequently are available in jails) and, therefore, decrease the risk of FAS or the severity of damage already incurred. However, there is evidence of unintended consequences with negative implications for prenatal care and birth outcome that make these actions problematic solutions to a medical and public health problem. Women who abuse illegal substances and who know that contact with health care systems might reveal this drug use and lead to incarceration or to removal of children from their care generally do not stop abusing, they simply do not seek medical care (Blume, in press; Geshan, 1993). Because alcohol is a legal substance, there have been fewer attempts at using such measures with women at risk for FAS. At least one Native American community has used tribal laws to allow for the enforced incarceration of pregnant women at very high risk for FAS. Treating a medical problem within the criminal justice system is unpalatable to the committee and viewed as highly unlikely to be effective. Mandated treatment for alcohol abuse in a therapeutic environment is a very different situation that has been debated for possible merits and many problems (Chavkin, 1991). At the simplest level, care that does not exist cannot be mandated. Many authors have documented the lack of treatment slots for pregnant women. Both the American Medical Association and the College of Obstetricians and Gynecologists oppose this approach.

Treatment of Alcohol Abuse and Dependence in Pregnant Women

For the comparatively small group of women who continue to abuse alcohol during pregnancy, formal treatment of alcohol dependence may be needed. There are a number of descriptions of comprehensive clinical treatment for pregnant alcohol-dependent women (Finkelstein, 1993; Jessup and Green, 1987; Rosett and Weiner, 1981a). The treatment programs described are typically broad, multimodal interventions that are intended to address the complex problems exhibited by this population. Thus, recommended treatments usually encompass medical and obstetric services, as well as alcohol and drug abuse services in the form of individual or group counseling, family therapy, referral to self-help groups, education about alcohol effects, parenting skills training, and case management. As mentioned earlier in this report, however, systematic data collection on characteristics of women who abuse alcohol during pregnancy has been rare. Thus, treatment programs for pregnant alcohol abusers have been based primarily on the availability of services and on clinical judgment, and in the relative absence of empirical data that could inform the conceptualization and development of treatments targeted to address the specific problems of this population.

Moreover, there are no data from randomized clinical trials evaluating treatment programs specifically for pregnant alcohol abusing women. Thus, the treatment packages or program components for pregnant alcohol abusers that have been described or implemented have not been evaluated specifically for (1) their ability to attract and retain pregnant women, (2) the impact of treatment programs or specific program components on maternal drinking behavior and related outcomes, or (3) the impact of these programs on infant outcomes. Similarly, there are no data from controlled trials on the optimal setting for such interventions (e.g., obstetrics-gynecology versus substance abuse treatment settings); the optimal intensity of treatment programs (e.g., hospital versus outpatient); the optimal duration of treatment; comparative effectiveness of alternate treatment approaches; and the relative efficacy of mixed- or single-gender programs.

Another barrier to evaluating the effectiveness of alcohol treatment for pregnant women is the paucity of appropriate services. For example, Chavkin and Kandall (1990) reported that 54 percent of drug treatment programs surveyed in New York City refused to accept pregnant women. Although several programs have been described and there have been a number of recent federal and state efforts to provide or expand treatment services for alcohol- and drug-abusing women, treatment programs may not be readily available to many of the women at risk.

Treatment Outcome Research on Alcohol Abuse in Women

The lack of data on effectiveness of treatment for pregnant women who abuse alcohol parallels the need for more data on the effectiveness of treatment for women who abuse alcohol in general. Most alcohol treatment outcome studies have been done with predominantly male samples. Vanicelli (1984) reported that in 530 treatment evaluation studies conducted between 1952 and 1980, only 7 percent of the subjects were women. A more recent review (Toneatto et al., 1992) of 108 treatment outcome studies states that many studies that could report outcome by gender do not do so; among those that have, there is no consistent evidence pointing to gender differences in outcome. Given the low number of women in most treatment outcome studies, it is unlikely that such studies would have the power to detect significant differences in outcome by gender. The low number of women included in most treatment outcome studies also limits the generalizability of findings to other samples of substance-abusing women. Furthermore, in cases where gender differences in treatment outcome are found, it is often unclear whether those differences are due to gender or are more directly associated with other prognostic factors that may vary with gender (e.g., SES, psychiatric disorders, marital status, age of onset).

Several important questions regarding treatment effectiveness for substance abusing women have not been addressed. There is at this time no strong evidence of gender differences in the determinants of treatment seeking, treatment retention, or outcome (IOM, 1990; McLellan et al., 1994); of modalities that may be better for women than for men; or of relative relapse in female versus male substance abusers. Research has not evaluated whether the multicomponent package approaches commonly recommended for substance-abusing women are more effective than unimodal approaches, although one controlled trial has suggested better outcomes for women in a single-gender program than in a mixed-gender program (Dahlgren and Willander, 1989). It should be noted that treatment content, duration, and intensity have not been well specified in many of these studies (e.g., through specification of treatments and monitoring of treatment implementation). It has therefore been difficult to evaluate systematically whether particular types of treatment, or treatment components, may be better for women than men.

Given a lack of strong evidence of the differential effectiveness of treatment for women and men at this time, treatment approaches that have been demonstrated to be effective for broad clinical populations could also be effective for women at risk for delivering infants with FAS, ARBD, or ARND. However, the effectiveness of approaches that have been evaluated primarily in nonfemale samples for women drinkers or women at risk for delivering infants with FAS, ARBD, or ARND should not be assumed. It should also be noted that at present there is no single treatment with demonstrated superiority of effectiveness for alcohol abuse (IOM, 1990; Miller and Hester, 1986). This implies the need for research on the applicability to pregnant alcohol abusers of a range of treatments with demonstrated effectiveness in the general clinical population. Strategies that have empirical support among clinical samples of alcohol-abusing individuals and may warrant evaluation as treatment for women at risk of delivering infants with FAS, ARBD, or ARND are reviewed briefly below, in order of intensity of treatment services. A model of treatment for pregnant women whose drinking puts them at risk for delivering an FAS infant may be stepped care, in which programs include a broad range of treatment intensities, from brief outpatient treatment to intensive residential treatment.

As discussed earlier, there is good evidence for the effectiveness of relatively low-cost, brief treatment approaches (Holder et al., 1991; IOM, 1990), such as motivational interviewing (Miller and Rollnick, 1991), for the treatment of alcohol abuse and dependence. These approaches attempt to mobilize the individual's own motivational resources to reduce or eliminate drinking. A feature that may make these approaches particularly appealing as a first-line intervention for women at risk of delivering FAS or ARBD infants is that they can be delivered in medical settings, where some women at risk may present (reviewed in Babor, 1994).

Cognitive-behavioral interventions, grounded in social learning theory, seek to impart generalizable coping skills that can be applied to reduce drinking and related problems. These approaches may be particularly promising for pregnant substance-abusing women in that they are geared to many of the problems noted among this population, including the use of alcohol and drugs in response to stress, lack of assertiveness and self-esteem, and links between psychiatric problems and substance use (IOM, 1990; Kadden et al., 1989).

Behavioral strategies, particularly those that seek to reinforce abstinence with positive incentives (e.g., Higgins et al., 1993, 1994; Stitzer et al., 1993) and those that address broad social problems (e.g., the community reinforcement approach), have been shown to be effective in retaining patients and reducing substance use in general clinical populations. Because these treatments can be tailored to target clearly defined outcomes (e.g., reductions in drinking, compliance with prenatal care), they could be adapted and evaluated among women at risk for delivering FAS infants.

Other, more intensive approaches, which have received little empirical evaluation but which have intuitive appeal for this population, should be evaluated. For example, although self-help groups, particularly Alcoholics Anonymous (AA), have been perceived as male oriented, evidence suggests that women may be more likely than men to attend self-help groups (Humphrey et al., 1991). The high level of social support provided in self-help groups and the recent development of specialized women's groups may make this a good option for pregnant women who abuse alcohol.

The most intensive level of care, that is, inpatient, residential, and day-treatment programs will be indicated for a proportion of pregnant alcohol-abusing women, particularly those with severe or refractory alcohol dependence, inadequate personal or financial resources, or severe comorbid psychopathology. These programs offer more structured and stable environments in which indicated medical and substance abuse treatment, as well as evaluation of related psychosocial problems, can be instituted. As noted, these important resources are still rare.

Addressing Barriers to Research

The lack of controlled trials of treatments for pregnant women at risk for delivering FAS infants highlights the many challenges involved in conducting this type of research. However, these challenges can be met, and systematic controlled evaluation of treatments for pregnant substance-abusing women is not impossible (Carroll et al., 1995) and should be pursued. Ideally, systematic evaluation of well-specified treatment programs for pregnant alcohol abusers should be undertaken for the many specialized programs now being implemented; this should then be followed by randomized controlled trials that rigorously evaluate the most promising approaches. Program evaluations and controlled trials should include methodological features that are increasingly standard in alcohol treatment efficacy research, including careful description of the study sample on clinically important dimensions, use of standardized assessment instruments to characterize the study sample and evaluate outcomes, careful specification of all aspects of study treatments in manuals, and clear definition of target outcomes.

Methodological and ethical issues involved in program evaluation and clinical trials of treatment for pregnant substance-abusing women are complex for many reasons. First, clinical research involving controlled or comparison designs requires careful consideration of ethical issues, particularly control conditions, because it would be unethical in most cases to randomize pregnant, treatment-seeking women to no-treatment conditions. However, it would be possible to compare well-defined multimodal approaches to minimal "standard" treatments, to study the components of treatment packages, and to evaluate the benefit of adding single innovative interventions to existing treatments. Second, investigators must carefully work through issues of confidentiality and protection of the women who agree to participate, as well as of their children. Third, as acknowledged earlier, the number of women at risk for delivering FAS infants is low; the number involved at any one time in a treatment program who are willing to participate in a randomized trial is likely to be even lower. Researchers interested in evaluating programs will thus be faced with the need to develop novel and active recruitment strategies and to consider the evaluation of women at risk in several sites. Because of the likely limitations on sample size, it may be necessary to report effect sizes rather than traditional measures of statistical significance.

MAINTENANCE AND AFTERCARE

Equally important to getting a pregnant woman who abuses alcohol to stop drinking is to keep her abuse under control after delivery. This will serve not only as prevention of FAS in future pregnancies, but also to improve the health and well-being of the mother, the newborn child, and any other children in the family. The literature in recent years suggests that an effective way to help alcohol-abusing women who had FAS children is through intensive case management (Bacon, 1988; Davis and Frost, 1984; Masis and May, 1991; Rosett and Weiner, 1981b; Weiner et al., 1989). Continuation of care into the post-partum period achieves or facilitates many goals. For example, this can eliminate the presence of alcohol in breast milk. It is standard medical advice that women who are breast-feeding not drink, which could further expose the infant to alcohol. Case management of women who have had one or more FAS children can help protect against further FAS children; help maintain better health status; coordinate substance abuse care throughout various institutions and agencies; and tailor care to specific social and medical needs of the woman, her family, and her children. Case management involves all members of the extended family and should include enlisting the positive action of the male partner. Children benefit from such efforts, too. Often children of FAS-producing mothers are in foster placement because of neglect or abuse. A major motivator for maintenance and aftercare is to improve the social and health status of the mother so that she can regain or retain custody of her children. Case management is also vital for FAS children. These children need a variety of services such as special education, special medical procedures, living assistance, behavioral therapy, and physical therapy. Many of these services will be needed throughout life (Dorris, 1989; Streissguth et al., 1986; Streissguth et al., 1991). This subject is discussed in Chapter 8.

An example of a case management approach is the Birth to Three Project in Seattle (Streissguth et al., 1993). Using existing services within a community, advocates work actively with each client to develop goals important to the woman herself. Postpartum women recruited into the program are those considered at the highest risk based on abuse of alcohol or other drugs during pregnancy, little or no prenatal care, and a lack of successful involvement with social service agencies. Important issues addressed initially include stable housing, substance abuse treatment with follow-up, health care, legal problems, and child custody. Longer-term issues include vocational and educational training, parenting skills, and social competence. The program was estimated to be very cost-effective.

PROGRAM EVALUATION

Prevention and treatment programs in all areas of substance abuse are infrequently evaluated, and rigorous evaluation is rare. For example, the Pregnant and

Post Partum Women and Their Infants (PPWI) program, administered by Substance Abuse and Mental Health Service Administration (SAMHSA) with funds contributed also by the Maternal and Child Health Bureau (MCHB) of Health Resources and Services Administration (HRSA), sponsored 147 demonstration-type programs for substance-abusing pregnant or postpartum women (National Center for Education in Maternal and Child Health, 1993). The types of interventions used in these programs were common sense approaches that seem, on consideration, to be reasonable. However, the program evaluation components are typically weak. For example, only half of the projects in existence in fiscal year 1993 had any type of evaluation. Most of these were pre- and posttest assessments of knowledge, attitudes, and beliefs. Of those, only half had a comparison group. Of those with a comparison group, a common comparison was with women who refused to participate in the program. Obviously, these programs provide important services to women in need but contribute little to a firm understanding of whether a program of interventions is effective at improving maternal and infant outcome or not.

Setting up an FAS prevention initiative with programmatic goals and objectives will facilitate evaluation of programs with multiple outcome measures, e.g., maternal outcome such as reducing alcohol consumption and infant outcome such as birth weight or FAS symptoms. Many prevention activities are evaluated for process outcomes only. In these cases, FAS is not the outcome measure. Rather, process evaluations focus on the number of women who enroll in the program, how many complete the program, and the like. The outcome measure of prime importance, however, would be changes in the incidence of FAS. Establishing the baseline prevalence of FAS in a community is the ideal first step in directly assessing the outcome of prevention efforts (May and Hymbaugh, 1983; May et al., 1983; Plaisier, 1989). This is a difficult outcome measure to use for several reasons. First, FAS is not very common. As described in Chapters 4 and 5, FAS is frequently difficult to diagnose except by highly trained persons. Thus, only large prevention programs with solid financial resources to include assessment by trained medical personnel would be able to detect changes in FAS incidence.

Therefore, proxy measures must frequently be used. As described in Chapter 5, proxy measures of infant outcome could be used. These might include the components most recognizable or easy to measure of the FAS diagnosis, such as head circumference or birth weight. Measuring knowledge gain and retention (Little et al., 1981, 1983; May and Hymbaugh, 1989), opinion and attitude changes, and surveys of behavior change all are possible proxy measures of success or failure in maternal outcome. However, they frequently represent measures of success with that part of the population at least risk for FAS, the moderate or minimal drinkers. For those at high risk, changes in relevant behavior are the most reasonable proxy measures. Thus, levels of drinking during pregnancy must be assessed reliably and routinely. Research is needed to suggest the most sensitive and cost-effective proxy measures of FAS for these purposes.

PUBLIC HEALTH SERVICE-FUNDED RESEARCH

The National Institute of Alcohol Abuse and Alcoholism (NIAAA) funds or has funded several projects that would provide fundamental information necessary for the design of prevention intervention projects (e.g., on health beliefs and knowledge about alcohol use in pregnancy, the impact of alcohol warning labels, the development of laboratory tests to detect alcohol abuse). Many of the projects funded through the NIAAA alcohol and pregnancy program are more basic studies using animal models or human in vitro methods. The importance and utility of these clinical and animal studies is explained throughout the report. The mainstays of clinical research projects have been the long-term follow-up studies of alcohol exposure during pregnancy (i.e., the Cleveland, Pittsburgh, Seattle, Detroit, and Atlanta projects referred to repeatedly in the text of this report). These projects have provided much important information used for diagnosis and for the epidemiologic study of the effects of less than heavy alcohol consumption. Identifying women who have given birth to a child affected by alcohol, even if not affected by FAS, ARBD, or ARND, is an important component of indicated prevention efforts.

Other programs within NIAAA provide or could provide information potentially relevant to FAS prevention. For example, many of the prevention and treatment projects aimed at alcohol abuse in general, and epidemiological studies of women in the general population, might provide information translatable to pregnant women. Most of the prevention and treatment projects, however, as pointed out in the previous section, do not currently focus on pregnant women or even on women. Nevertheless, NIAAA-funded research has elucidated fundamentals of alcohol abuse prevention and treatment in general, and some projects funded in the future could focus on or at least include women and pregnant women.

Several of the CDC state-based prevention projects are involved in what the committee would consider universal prevention activities. The Colorado project is embarking on developing statewide media campaigns about FAS. The Alaska project is identifying statewide information and awareness needs about FAS and is working to identify how prepared health care providers feel about discussing alcohol issues with patients, including their comfort level with referring those in need for treatment. FAS workers in Oklahoma are developing and implementing education programs about FAS targeted to health care providers. The project in South Dakota, which is conducted in conjunction with the Indian Health Service, is working to change community attitudes toward drinking during pregnancy. There are currently no firm data from any of these projects with which to ascertain their effectiveness—data that are crucial for decisionmakers who need to prioritize their increasingly sparse public health prevention resources.

Several of the CDC state and university projects involve activities that the committee would consider selective interventions. Many (e.g., Colorado, Kansas, and South Dakota) are explicitly working on identification of women at risk for substance abuse. The projects in Georgia, Colorado, and Oklahoma include the development of training materials for professionals to identify women at high risk for FAS. Two demonstration projects in Missouri offer alcohol education to high-risk women (i.e., women encountered in the Division of Family Services Alternate Care Program). The Missouri project will also offer family planning services to women in substance abuse treatment programs. The University of Cincinnati project is using a randomized controlled methodology comparing standard care versus intensive, prenatal intervention with pregnant drinkers. The outcome measures in this project will include maternal and infant characteristics.

The committee identified at least two CDC FAS prevention projects that are involved in gathering fundamental information relevant for what the committee defines as indicated prevention programs. The Alaska project is examining the social, medical, and reproductive histories of women who have given birth to at least one FAS child. The data could then be used as a framework for developing interventions aimed at these highest-risk mothers. The state-based program in Washington also includes efforts to identify characteristics of the biological mothers of FAS children and to identify, locate, track, and follow-up the biological mothers of children identified in the University of Washington FAS clinic.

SUMMARY

The detailed prevention measures described above represent a progression through a spectrum. Universal prevention is used to promote general knowledge and social conditions that serve to reduce substance abuse and to promote healthy pregnancy practices. Selective prevention targets groups that include people at risk. Indicated prevention is applied to individuals identified as at risk for adverse outcomes. The effects of heavy and persistent alcohol abuse on pregnancy are already established. If a woman or couple has diagnosed problems of alcohol or substance abuse, specific steps, indicated prevention action, must be taken to break the causal chain and to adapt to the needs and problems created by the maternal behavior. Such treatment steps for the mother are preventive for FAS.

The women who drink most heavily are the least likely to lower their alcohol consumption on their own during pregnancy, and they compromise their own welfare as well as the well-being of the larger community (May, 1991). Women who continue to participate in substance abuse and risky pregnancy practices, despite attempts at motivation and empathic approaches to change, are candidates for very intensive treatment.

At advanced stages of heavy drinking and alcohol abuse, a woman may no longer be able to control her own health status (due to social, economic, medical, and psychological barriers). For such a woman, treatment for alcohol abuse as a means to prevent FAS could also be a means to enhance her ability to reduce her disability and to reenter a state of health, healthy behavior, and mainstream society. Many women who drink heavily are ostracized, which may discourage their entry into treatment or reentry to mainstream society (Blume, in press; May et al., 1983). The indicated level of prevention, alcohol treatment, and mainte-nance, when facilitated by well-trained case managers, can provide such a ve-hicle. If one wants to reduce the prevalence of FAS in a short period of time, using case-managers to institute indicated prevention, treatment, and aftercare might effect such change (Masis and May, 1991).

Recent studies show that while approximately 20 percent of all women continue to drink during pregnancy, most women reduce their consumption dur-ing pregnancy. Furthermore, women who abuse alcohol are a small subset of drinking women (Grant et al., 1994; Serdula et al., 1991). Therefore, indicated prevention, treatment, and aftercare are considered necessary only for a small proportion of the population.

RECOMMENDATIONS

• The committee recommends that until such time as clear dose-response relationships are established, pregnant women and those about to become preg-nant be counseled to avoid alcohol consumption throughout pregnancy.

• The committee recommends greatly increased attention among sponsors of prevention initiatives, independent of the target population, to evaluating the effectiveness of programs implemented. This recommendation applies to all levels of prevention interventions.

• The committee recommends that research efforts include comparisons of prevention methods at all levels in order to provide information to policy makers about relative costs and benefits.

Indicated prevention interventions:

• The committee recommends that a high priority be placed on research efforts to design, implement, and evaluate prevention interventions that can ef-fectively guide pregnant women who drink heavily to alcohol treatment. Re-search or programs should also include:

— implementation of appropriate screening tools, including bio-markers of alcohol exposure, to identify women who are drinking moderate to heavy amounts of alcohol during pregnancy;

— assessment of methods to involve women's partners and family members in interventions to decrease or stop drinking;

— incorporation of comprehensive reproductive counseling and contraceptive services in prevention and treatment programs for substance-abusing women;

— assessment of the effectiveness and economic benefits of protocols for case management and follow-up of women, and of their families, who have given birth to a child affected by fetal alcohol exposure;

— development of training programs for professionals in the identification of heavy drinking, and referral to appropriate regional centers or prevention services;

— use of multiple outcome measures to assess the effectiveness of prevention initiatives; and

— basic research in animal models to elucidate further the mechanisms of alcohol teratogenesis, which might lead to pharmacologic or other strategies for amelioration of the effects of alcohol exposure in utero.

Selective prevention interventions:

• The committee recommends increased research efforts to design, implement, and evaluate selective prevention interventions to decrease risks of FAS, ARND, and ARBD through programs aimed toward women who are pregnant or may become pregnant, and who drink alcohol. Designing such interventions will be aided by further research assessing the contribution of personal and socio-environmental risk and protective factors that affect levels of drinking by women during pregnancy.

• Where the utility of specific intervention programs has been established, the committee recommends broad implementation of successful prevention interventions. Programs developed or studied should include the following:

— specific demographic groups that have been demonstrated to be at higher risk for FAS, ARBD, and ARND, as well as those who exhibit risk factors associated with moderate to heavy alcohol consumption during pregnancy; and

— implementation of prevention efforts in a wide range of communities and media;

Universal prevention interventions:

• The committee recommends that although data are insufficient regarding the effectiveness of universal prevention interventions, such interventions should be continued to raise awareness about the risks of FAS, ARBD, and ARND. However, the most important approach to universal prevention is probably the development of a medical environment in which concepts of the risk of FAS, ARBD, and ARND are incorporated into routine health care. Further education efforts to reach children and adults about FAS, ARBD, and ARND through health educational curricula and other means are recommended.

REFERENCES

Abel EL. Marihuana, Tobacco, Alcohol, and Reproduction. Boca Raton, FL: CRC Press, 1983.

Abel EL. Fetal alcohol syndrome in families (Commentary). Neurotoxicology and Teratology 1988; 10:12.

Abel EL. Rat offspring aired by males treated with alcohol. Alcohol 1993; 10:237-242.

Abel EL, Bilitzke PB. Paternal alcohol exposure: Paradoxical effect in mice and rats. Psychopharmacology 1990; 100:159-164.

Abel EL, Sokol RJ. Maternal and fetal characteristics affecting alcohol's teratogenicity. Neurobehavioral Toxicology and Teratology 1986; 8:329-334.

Abel EL, Tan SE. Effects of paternal alcohol consumption on pregnancy outcome in rats. Neurotoxicology and Teratology 1986; 10:167-192.

Addiction Research Foundation of Ontario, Canadian Centre on Substance Abuse. Appendix 1—Moderate drinking and health: A joint policy statement based on the International Symposium on Moderate Drinking and Health, April 30-May 1, 1993, in Toronto, Canada. Canadian Medical Association Journal 1994; 151:821-824.

Adger H, McDonald EM, DeAngelis C. Substance abuse education in pediatrics. Pediatrics 1990; 86:555-560.

American College of Obstetricians and Gynecologists. Substance Abuse in Pregnancy. ACOG Technical Bulletin 195:1994.

American Psychiatric Association. Diagnostic and Statistical Manual of Mental Disorders: 3rd Edition. Washington, DC: APA, 1980.

Anton RF, Moak DH. Carbohydrate-deficient transferrin and γ-glutamyltransferase as markers of heavy alcohol consumption: gender differences. Alcoholism: Clinical and Experimental Research 1994; 18:747-754.

Ashley MJ, Ferrence R, Room R, Rankin J, Single E. Moderate drinking and health: Report of an international symposium. Canadian Medical Association Journal 1994; 151:809-828.

Babor TF. Avoiding the horrid and beastly sin of drunkenness: Does dissuasion make a difference? Journal of Consulting and Clinical Psychology 1994; 62:1127-1140.

Bacon FS. Counseling aspects of alcohol use in pregnancy—Beyond primary prevention. Alcoholism treatment quarterly 1988; 5:257-267.

Bingol N, Schuster C, Fuchs J, Iosub S, Turner G, Stone RK et al. Influence of socio-economic factors on the occurrence of Fetal Alcohol Syndrome. Advances in Alcohol and Substance Abuse 1987; 6:105-118.

Bloom M. Primary Prevention: The Possible Science. Englewood Cliffs, New Jersey: Prentice-Hall, Inc., 1981.

Blume SB. Women and Alcohol: Issues in Social Policy in Alcohol and Gender. R. W. Wilsnack and S. C. Wilsnack (eds.). New Brunswick, New Jersey: Rutgers University Center of Alcohol Studies, in press.

Bowen OR, Sammons JH. The alcohol-abusing patient: A challenge to the profession. Journal of the American Medical Association 1988; 260:2267-2270.

Bradley KA, Larson EB. Training physicians to help patients who drink too much [editorial; comment]. Journal of General Internal Medicine 1994; 9:296-298.

Brown RT, Coles CD, Smith IE, Platzman KA, Silverstein J, Erickson S et al. Effects of prenatal alcohol exposure at school age. II. Attention and behavior. Neurotoxicology and Teratology 1991; 13:369-376.

Carroll KD, Change G, Behr H, Clinton B, Kosten TR. Improving treatment outcome in pregnant methadone-maintained women: Results from a randomized clinical trial. American Journal on Addictions 1995; 4:56-59.

Casswell S, Gilmore L. An evaluated community action project on alcohol. Journal of Studies in Alcohol 1989; 50:339-346.

Cefalo RC, Moos MK. Preconceptional Health: A Practical Guide. St. Louis: Mosby, 1995.

Centers for Disease Control and Prevention. Update: Trends in fetal alcohol syndrome—United States, 1979-1993. Morbidity and Mortality Weekly Report 1995a;44:249-251.

Centers for Disease Control and Prevention. Sociodemographic and behavioral characteristics associated with alcohol consumption during pregnancy—United States, 1988. MMWR 1995b; 44:261-264.

Chavkin W. Mandatory treatment for drug use during pregnancy. Journal of the American Medical Association 1991; 266:1556-1561.

Chavkin W, Kandall SR. Between a "Rock" and a hard place: Perinatal drug abuse. Pediatrics 1990; 85:223-225.

Cicero TJ. Effects of paternal exposure to alcohol on offspring development. Alcohol Health & Research World 1994; 18:37-41.

Clarren SK. Recognition of fetal alcohol syndrome. Journal of the American Medical Association 1981; 245:2436-2439.

Coles CD, Smith IE, Fernhoff PM, Falek A. Neonatal ethanol withdrawal: Characteristics in clinically normal, nondysmorphic neonates. Journal of Pediatrics 1984; 105:445-451.

Coles CD, Smith I, Fernhoff PM, Falek A. Neonatal neurobehavioral characteristics as correlates of maternal alcohol use during gestation. Alcoholism: Clinical and Experimental Research 1985; 9:454-460.

Coles CD, Smith IE, Lancaster JS, Falek A. Persistence over the first month of neurobehavioral alterations in infants exposed to alcohol prenatally. Infant Behavior and Development 1987; 10:23-37.

Coles CD, Brown RT, Smith IE, Platzman KA, Erickson S, Falek A. Effects of prenatal alcohol exposure at 6 years: I. Physical and cognitive development. Neurotoxicology 1991; 13:1-11.

Davis A, Lipson A. A challenge in managing a family with Fetal Alcohol Syndrome. Clinical Pediatrics 1984; 23:304.

Davis JH, Frost WA. Fetal Alcohol Syndrome: A challenge for the community health nurse. Journal of Community Health Nursing 1984; 1:99-110.

Day NL, Cottreau CM, Richardson GA. The epidemiology of alcohol, marijuana, and cocaine use among women of childbearing age and pregnant women. Clinical Obstetrics and Gynecology 1993; 36:232-245.

Day NL, Robles N, Richardson G, Geva D, Taylor P, Scher M et al. The effects of prenatal alcohol use in the growth of children at three years of age. Alcoholism: Clinical and Experimental Research 1991; 15:67-71.

Day N, Richardson G, Robles N et al. Effect of prenatal alcohol exposure on growth and morphology of the offspring at age three. Poster presented at ISBRA/RSA Congress, June 17-22, 1990, Toronto, Canada.

Dahlgren L, Willander A. Are special facilities for female alcoholics needed? A controlled 2-year follow-up study from a specialized female unit (EWA) versus a mixed male/female treatment facility. Alcoholism: Clinical and Experimental Research 1989; 11:499-504.

Dorris M. The Broken Cord. New York: Harper & Row, 1989.

Dufour MC, Williams GD, Campbell KE, Aitken SS. Knowledge of FAS and the risks of heavy drinking during pregnancy, 1985 and 1990 [NIAAA's Epidemiologic Bulletin No. 33]. Alcohol Health & Research World 1994; 18:86-92.

Ewing JA. Detecting alcoholism: The CAGE questionnaire. Journal of the American Medical Association 1984; 252:1905-1907.

Faden VB, Graubard BI, Dufour M. Drinking by expectant mothers—What does it mean for their babies? Working paper, Division of Biometry and Epidemiology, National Institute on Alcohol Abuse and Alcoholism 1994.

Faden VB, Hanna EZ. Alcohol and pregnancy—To drink or not to drink? Paper Presented at the Conference on Psychosocial and Behavioral Factors in Women's Health. American Psychological Association, Washington, DC 1994.

Fetal Alcohol Prevention and Education Family Album, Developed by the Spokane Tribe of Indians Fetal Alcohol Program; Spokane Tribal Community Action Team, Wellpinit, Washington.

Finkelstein N. Treatment programming for alcohol and drug-dependent pregnant women. International Journal of the Addictions 1993; 28:1275-1309.

Fitzgerald P. FAS persists despite broad public awareness. Michigan Medicine 1988; May, 262-268.

Fuchs CW, Stampfer MD, Colditz GA, Giovannucci EL, Manson JE, Kawachi I et al. Alcohol consumption and mortality among women. New England Journal of Medicine 1995; 19:1245-1250.

Galanter M. (ed.) Recent Developments in Alcoholism. Volume XII: Alcoholism in Women: The effect of gender. New York: Plenum, in press.

Geshan S. A Step Toward Recovery: Improving Access to Substance Abuse Treatment for Pregnant and Parenting Women. DC: Southern Regional Project on Infant Mortality, 1993.

Gjerde H, Johnson J, Bjorneboe A, Bjorneboe GEA, Morland J. A comparison of serum carbohydrate-deficient transferrin with other biological markers of excessive drinking. Scandinavian Journal of Clinical Laboratory Investigation 1988; 48:106.

Gomberg ESL, Nirenberg RD (eds.). Women and Substance Abuse. Norwood, New Jersey: Ablex, 1993.

Gordon RS, Jr. An operations classification of disease prevention. Public Health Reports 1983; 98:107-109.

Gordon R. An Operational Classification of Disease Prevention. Preventing Mental Disorders. J. A. Steinberg and M. M. Silverman (eds.). Rockville, MD: National Institute of Mental Health, 1987.

Grant BF, Harford TC, Dawson DA, Chou P, DuFour M, Pickering R. Prevalence of DSM-IV alcohol abuse and dependence United States, 1992. Alcohol Health and Research World 1994; 18:243-248.

Halvorson MR, Campbell JL, Sprague G, Slater K, Noffsinger JK, Peterson CM. Comparative evaluation of the clinical utility of three markers of ethanol intake: The effect of gender. Alcoholism: Clinical and Experimental Research 1993a; 17:225.

Halvorson MR, Noffsinger JK, Peterson CM. Studies of whole blood-associated acetaldehyde levels in teetotalers. Alcohol 1993b; 19:409-413.

Hankin JR. FAS prevention strategies: Passive and active measures. Alcohol Health & Research World 1994; 18:62-66.

Harouki R, Chobert MN, Finidori J, Aggerbeck M, Nalpas B, Hanoune J. Ethanol effects in a rat hepatoma cell line: Induction of gamma glutamyl transferase. Hepatology 1983; 3:323-329.

Hazlett LD, Barrett RP, Berk RS, Abel EL. Maternal and paternal alcohol consumption increase offspring susceptibility to P. aeruginosa ocular infection. Ophthalmic Research 1989; 21:381-387.

Higgins ST, Budney AJ, Bickel WK, Hughes JR. Achieving cocaine abstinence with a behavioral approach. American Journal of Psychiatry 1993; 150:763-769.

Higgins ST, Budney AJ, Bickel WK, Foerg FE, Donham R, Budger GJ. Incentives improve outcome in out-patient behavioral treatment of cocaine dependence. Archives of General Psychiatry 1994; 51:568-576.

Holder HD, Longabaugh R, Miller WR, Robonis AV. The cost effectiveness of treatment for alcohol problems: A first approximation. Journal of Studies on Alcohol 1991; 52:517-540.

Humphrey K, Marvis B, Stofflemavr B. Factors predicting attendance at self-help after substance abuse treatment: Preliminary findings. Journal of Consulting and Clinical Psychology 1991; 59:591-593.

Institute of Medicine. Broadening the Base of Treatment of Alcohol Problems. Washington, DC: National Academy Press, 1990.

Institute of Medicine. Disability in American. Washington, DC: National Academy Press, 1991.

Institute of Medicine. Reducing Risks for Mental Disorders: Frontiers for Prevention Intervention Research. Washington, DC: National Academy Press, 1994.

Institute of Medicine. The Best Intentions: Unintended Pregnancy and the Well-Being of Children and Families. Washington, DC: National Academy Press, 1995.

Jacob T., Premer DA. Assortive mating among men and women alcoholics. Journal of Studies on Alcohol 1986; 47:219-222.

Jacobson JL, Jacobson SW. Prenatal alcohol exposure and neurobehavioral development: Where is the Threshold? Alcohol Health & Research World—[Special Focus: Alcohol-Related Birth Defects]. Dianne M. Welsh (ed.). 18. Rockville, MD: National Institute on Alcohol Abuse and Alcoholism: 1994:30-36.

Jessup M, Green JR. Treatment of the pregnant alcohol-dependent woman. Journal of Psychoactive Drugs 1987; 19:193-203.

Kadden RM, Cooney NL, Getter H, Litt M. Matching alcoholics to coping skills or interactional therapies: Posttreatment results. Journal of Consulting and Clinical Psychology 1989; 57:698-704.

Korri UM, Nuutinen H, Salaspuro M. Increased blood acetate: A new laboratory marker of alcoholism and heavy drinking. Alcoholism: Clinical and Experimental Research 1985; 9:468-471.

Little R, Grathwohl HL, Streissguth AP, McIntyre C. Public knowledge about the risks of drinking during pregnancy in Multnomah County, Oregon. American Journal of Public Health 1981; 71:312-314.

Little RE, Streissguth AP, Guzenski GM, Grathwohl HL, Blumhagne JM, McIntyre CE. Change in obstetrician advice following a two-year community educational program on alcohol use and pregnancy. American Journal of Obstetrics and Gynecology 1983; 146:23-28.

Masis KB, May PA. A comprehensive local program for the prevention of fetal alcohol syndrome. Public Health Reports 1991; 106:484-489.

Mausner JS, Kramer S. Epidemiology: An introductory text. Philadelphia: W. B. Saunders Co., 1985.

May PA. Fetal alcohol effects among North American Indians: Evidence and implications for society. Alcohol Health & Research World 1991; 15(3):239-248.

May PA. The epidemiology of alcohol abuse among American Indians: The mythical and real properties. Journal of American Indian Culture 1994; 18:121-143.

May PA. Research issues in the prevention of fetal alcohol syndrome (FAS) and alcohol-related birth defects (ARBD). Prevention Research on Women and Alcohol. E. Taylor, J. Howard, P. Mail, M. Hilton (eds.). Washington, DC: U.S. Government Printing Office, in press.

May PA, Hymbaugh KJ, Aase JM, Samet JM. Epidemiology of fetal alcohol syndrome among American Indians of the Southwest. Social Biology 1983; 30:374-387.

May PA, Hymbaugh KJ. A macro-level fetal alcohol syndrome prevention program for Native Americans and Alaska Natives: Description and evaluation. Journal of Studies on Alcoholism 1989; 50:508-518.

May PA, Hymbaugh KJ. A pilot project on fetal alcohol syndrome among American Indians. Alcohol Health & Research World 1983; 7:3-9.

McLellan AT, Alterman AI, Metzger DS, Grissom GR, Woody GE, Luborsky L, O'Brien CP. Similarity of outcome predictors across opiate, cocaine, and alcohol treatments: Role of treatment services. Journal of Consulting and Clinical Psychology 1994; 62:1141-1158.

Mihas AA, Tavassoli M. Laboratory markers of ethanol intake and abuse: A critical appraisal. American Journal of Medical Sciences 1992; 303:415-428.

Miller WR, Hester RK. The effectiveness of alcoholism treatment: What research reveals. Treating additive behaviors: Processes of change. W.R. Miller and R.K. Hester (eds.). New York: Plenum, 1986:121-174.

Miller WR, Rollnick S. Motivational interviewing: Preparing people to change addictive behavior. New York: Guilford, 1991.

Mosher JF, Jernigan DW. New directions in alcohol policy. Annual Review of Public Health 1989; 10:245-279.

Mullen PC, Glenday MA. Alcohol Avoidance Counseling in Prenatal Care. New Perspectives on Prenatal Care. I. R. Merkatz, J. E. Thompason (eds.), P. D. Mullen and R. L. Goldenberg, (Assoc. eds.). New York: Elsevier, 1990.

National Center for Education in Maternal and Child Health. Prevention of Perinatal Substance Use: Pregnant and Postpartum Women and Their Infants Demonstration Grant Program—Abstracts of Active Projects Fiscal Year 1993. Arlington, VA: National Center for Education in Maternal and Child Health. 1993.

National Institute on Alcohol Abuse and Alcoholism. Alcoholism and alcohol abuse among women: Research issues (NIAAA Research Monograph No. 1). Washington, DC: U. S. Department of Health, Education and Welfare (Publication No. ADM 80-835), 1980.

National Institute on Drug Abuse. NIDA survey examines extent of women's drug use during pregnancy. NIDA Media Advisory. Rockville, MD: NIDA, 1994.

Niemelä O, Halmemake E, Jlikorkala O. Hemoglobin-acetaldehyde adducts are elevated in women carrying alcohol-damaged fetuses. Alcohol: Clinical and Experimental Research 1991; 15:1007-1010.

Peterson CM, Ross SL, Scott BK. Correlation of self-administered alcoholism screening test with hemoglobin-associated acetaldehyde. Alcohol 1990; 7:289-293.

Plaisier KJ. Fetal alcohol syndrome prevention in American Indian communities of Michigan's upper peninsula. American Indian and Alaska Native Mental Health Research 1989; 3:16-33.

Rosett HL, Weiner L. Identifying and treating pregnant patients at risk from alcohol. Canadian Medical Journal 1981a; 125:149-154.

Rosett HL, Weiner L, Edelin KC. Strategies for prevention of fetal alcohol effects. Obstetrics and Gynecology 1981b; 57:1-7.

Russell M. Clinical implications of recent research on the fetal alcohol syndrome. Bulletin of the New York Academy of Medicine 1991; 67:207-222.

Russell M. New assessment tools for risk drinking during pregnancy. Alcohol Health and Research World 1994; 18:55-61.

Savitz DA, Schwingl PJ, Keels MA. Influence of paternal age, smoking, and alcohol consumption on congenital anomalies. Teratology 1991; 44:429-440.

Savitz DA, Zhang J, Schwingl P, John EM. Association of paternal alcohol use with gestational age and birth weight. Teratology 1992; 46:465-471.

Selzer ML. The Michigan Alcoholism Screening Test: The quest for a new diagnostic instrument. American Journal of Psychiatry 1971; 127:1653-1658.

Serdula M, Williamson DF, Kendrick JS, Anda RF, Byers T. Trends in alcohol consumption by pregnant women: 1985 through 1988. Journal of the American Medical Association 1991; 265:876-879.

Single E. The control of public drinking: The impact of the environment on alcohol problems. Control Issues in Alcohol Abuse Prevention: Strategies for States and Communities. H.D. Holder (ed.). Greenwich, CT: JAI Press, 1987.

Smith IE, Coles CD, Lancaster JS, Fernhoff PM, Falek A. The effect of volume and duration of prenatal ethanol exposure on neonatal physical and behavioral development. Neurobehavioral Toxicology and Teratology 1986;8:375-381.

Smith IE, Lancaster JS, Moss-Wells S, Coles CD, Falek A. Identifying high-risk pregnant drinkers: biological and behavioral correlates of continuous heavy drinking during pregnancy. Journal of Studies on Alcohol 1987; 48:304-309.

Sokol RJ, Martier SS, Ager JW. The T-ACE questions: Practical prenatal detection of risk-drinking. American Journal of Obstetrics and Gynecology 1989; 160:863-868.

Sokol RJ, Miller SI, Reed G. Alcohol abuse during pregnancy: An epidemiological study. Alcoholism: Clinical and Experimental Research 1980; 4:135-145.

Sokol RJ, Miller SI, Martier S. Identifying the alcohol-abusing obstetric/gynecologic patient: A practical approach. Washington, DC: U.S. Department of Health and Human Services, NIAAA, (Publication No. ADM 81-1163), 1991.

Stibler H, Borg S, Allgulander C. Clinical significance of abnormal microheterogeneity of transferrin in relation to alcohol consumption. Acta Medica Scandinavica 1979; 206:275-281.

Stitzer ML, Iguchi MY, Kidorf M, Bigelow GE. Contingency management in methadone treatment: The case for positive incentives. Behavioral treatments for drug abuse and dependence. L.S. Onken, J.D. Blaine, J.J. Boren (eds.). Rockville, Maryland: National Institute on Drug Abuse, 1993.

Storey EL, Anderson GJ, Mack U, Powell LW, Halliday JW. Desialylated transferrin as a serological marker of chronic excessive alcohol ingestion. Lancet 1987; 1:1292-1294.

Streissguth AP, Aase JM, Clarren SK, Randels SP, LaDue RA, Smith DF. Fetal alcohol syndrome in adolescents and adults. Journal of the American Medical Association 1991; 265:1961-1967.

Streissguth AP, Grant T, Ernst CC, Phipps P. Reaching out to the highest risk mothers: the Birth to 3 Project. Pregnancy & Health Studies, University of Washington, Seattle, Technical Report No. 93-02. April 27, 1993.

Streissguth AP, LaDue RA, Randels SP. A Manual on Adolescents and Adults with FAS with Special Reference to American Indians. Rockville, MD: U.S. Indian Health Service, 1986.

Toneatto A, Sobell LC, Sobell MB. Gender differences in the treatment of abusers of alcohol and other drugs. Journal of Substance Abuse 1992; 4:209-218.

U.S. Department of Health and Human Services, Public Health Service, Office of Disease Prevention and Health Promotion (ODPHP). Healthy People 2000: National Health Promotion and Disease Prevention Objectives. Conference Edition. U.S. DHHS: Washington, D.C., September 1990.

U.S. Department of Health and Human Services. Alcohol and Health [Eighth Special Report to the U.S. Congress]. Washington, DC: U.S. Department of Health and Human Services, 1993.

U.S. Public Health Service. Surgeon General's Advisory on Alcohol and Pregnancy. Food and Drug Administration Bulletin 1981; 11:9-10.

Vanicelli M. Treatment outcome of alcoholic women. The state of art in relation to sex bias and expectancy effects. Alcohol Problems in Women. S.C. Wilsnack and L.J. Beclanan (eds.). New York: Guilford, 1984:369-412.

Wallack L. Practical issues, ethical concerns and future directions in the prevention of alcohol-related problems. Journal of Primary Prevention 1984; 4:199-224.

Waterson EJ, Murray-Lyon IM. Alcohol, smoking and pregnancy: Some observations on ethnic minorities in the United Kingdom. British Journal of Addiction 1989; 84:323-325.

Waterson EJ, Murray-Lyon IM. Preventing alcohol related birth damage: A review. Social Science and Medicine 1990; 30:349-364.

Weiner L, Morse BA, Garrido P. FAS/FAE: Focusing prevention on women at risk. International Journal of the Addictions 1989; 24:385-395.

Wilsnack SC. Alcohol Use and Alcohol Problems in Women. Psychology of Women's Health: Progress and Challenges in Research and Application. A. L. Stanton and S. J. Gallant (eds.). Washington, DC: American Psychological Association, in press.

Wilsnack SC. Patterns and trends in women's drinking: Recent findings and some implications for prevention. Prevention Research on Women and Alcohol. E. Taylor, J. Howard, P. Mail, M. Hilton (eds.). Washington, DC: U.S. Government Printing Office, in press.

Wilsnack SC, Beckman LJ. Alcohol Problems in Women: Antecedents, Consequences, and Intervention. New York: Guilford Press, 1984.

Wilsnack SC, Klassen AD, Schur BE, Wilsnack RW. Predicting onset and chronicity of women's problem drinking: A five-year longitudinal analysis. American Journal of Public Health 1991; 81:305-318.

8

The Affected Individual: Clinical Presentation, Intervention, and Treatment

Despite the apparently large number of affected individuals who are born each year (see Chapter 5), fetal alcohol syndrome (FAS), alcohol-related birth defects (ARBD), and alcohol-related neurodevelopmental disorder (ARND) are rarely diagnosed. Similarly, although developmental problems in children have been demonstrated through prospective studies to be associated with maternal substance use (Streissguth et al., 1993), these problems are often not acknowledged except in the most extreme cases. Because of the difficulty in identification, as well as environmental factors, learning problems and aberrant behaviors can be attributed to other causes. As a result, many affected individuals do not receive correct diagnosis or treatment for their alcohol-related disabilities.

For obvious reasons, the focus of prevention efforts has been on the prevention of maternal alcohol use in pregnancy or on the prevention of pregnancy itself. The logic has been that such activities will be most cost-effective and, ultimately, have the greatest benefit for both mother and offspring. However, despite our best efforts (see Chapter 7), neither universal prevention nor more targeted activities have had a very strong impact on those persons most at risk (Smith and Coles, 1991), and many children are born affected by their teratogenic exposure. For these children, there has been a curious lack of enthusiasm for targeted efforts directed at the prevention of secondary disabilities. Such efforts might prevent some of the more negative outcomes reported to be associated with FAS (Dorris, 1989; Lemoine and Lemoine, 1992; Spohr et al., 1993).

Originally, it was not clear which factors produced these poor developmental outcomes—whether, that is, the observed problems resulted from damage to the nervous system or from poor caregiving. However, there are now convergent data from long-term clinical studies of individuals with FAS gathered from a number of different populations (Lemoine and Lemoine, 1992 [France]; Steinhausen et al., 1993 [Germany]; Streissguth et al., 1991 [Native American]) arguing that outcome can be predicted most effectively by examining the interaction between severity of biological insult (operationally defined as dysmorphia) and environmental risk (operationally defined as caregiving instability and abuse or neglect). This relationship comes as no surprise, because it is well known that in other studies of high-risk children, poor social and caregiving environments exacerbate negative outcomes, whereas middle-class social status (Aylward, 1992) and well-designed early intervention (Bryant and Ramey, 1987) ameliorate these negative effects. However, few systematic attempts have been made to intervene with alcohol-affected children to test the possibility that such strategies would be effective in producing more positive outcomes.

It is possible to speculate on reasons for the lack of interest in intervention with this group of children (see Coles and Platzman, 1992). Many of those identified as alcohol-affected are of minority or low socioeconomic status (SES) (Abel, 1995). For these reasons, families often lack the resources that are required to access appropriate services (Anderson and Novick, 1992). It is also well known that most medical and other professionals are not comfortable dealing with substance abuse or with addicts (Chappel, 1973; Robinson and Podnos, 1966). In addition, however, there has been an attitude that "the damage is done" and that, given the biological nature of the insult to the nervous system, there is little to be done to help affected children. Some clinical studies have appeared to suggest that an optimal rearing environment may not significantly alter the deficits observed in children with FAS (Streissguth et al., 1985). However, others have argued that postnatal environment and experience do, indeed, significantly influence outcome in terms of both behavioral and cognitive development (Brown et al., 1991; Smith and Coles, 1991). Although there are few clinical studies in affected children, animal research suggests that the postnatal rearing environment may have positive outcomes even in alcoholized animals (Hannigan et al., 1993; Weinberg et al., in press). Although one cannot extrapolate directly from findings in animals to the clinical setting, the present data certainly indicate one possible direction for future research on treatment of children exposed to alcohol prenatally.

When considered, the view that intervention may not be useful in children affected by alcohol seems odd, because it is inconsistent with the attitude taken toward other groups of high-risk and disabled children, who are the focus of many early intervention and special education efforts (Meisels and Shonkoff, 1990). Children with Down syndrome, for instance, usually are more seriously affected than those with FAS. Nevertheless, such children are regularly identified early and placed in intervention (Farran, 1990), although their developmental scores during the first year often do not qualify them for services.

There appear to be several kinds of barriers that have prevented alcohol-affected children from receiving appropriate intervention and treatment services. These problems may include the following: (1) The characteristics of the children themselves have not been well understood, so it has been difficult to understand how to intervene. (2) The nature of the insult to the developing child is such that, often, these children do not qualify for existing services. (3) Some services that might benefit mothers and children do not exist or are not widely available. (4) It is difficult for most professionals to deal with substance abuse due to lack of training, denial, and other social or emotional reactions. (5) There are many barriers to the interaction of the systems that serve children and those that serve recovering mothers so that the needs of the family often are overlooked (Coles and Platzman, 1992). These issues are explored in this chapter. The chapter begins with a description of clinical issues, including a description of what is currently know about the medical, behavioral, and social problems documented in people with FAS. These are discussed in a chronologic manner, beginning with infancy, in which most information has been gathered, and ending in adulthood, a period for which little information is available. Key questions about these issues that are relevant for planning interventions are described. The chapter then goes on to discuss what is known about interventions (medical, educational, and family-oriented initiatives) and the possibilities for decreasing secondary disabilities. The chapter concludes with a discussion on the limitations and barriers to the provision of services to people with FAS.

CLINICAL ISSUES IN INDIVIDUALS WITH FAS, ARBD, OR ARND

Medical Overview: FAS Health Issues

In general, children with fetal alcohol syndrome require little more than routine medical care. However, a number of physical problems have been reported to be related to alcohol exposure and should be considered specifically. These include cardiac defects, urogenital problems, skeletal abnormalities (Streissguth et al., 1985), visual problems (Stromland, 1981), hearing deficiencies (Church and Gerkin, 1988), and dental abnormalities (Barnett and Schusterman, 1985). Necessary attention to these problems varies with the age of the child.

In infancy, children with fetal alcohol syndrome should be carefully examined for associated major malformations. Associated defects of the heart and skeletal system can be excluded through a careful physical exam. Problems of the urogenital system, including hydronephrosis and kidney anomalies, cannot be excluded without imaging studies. Because no accurate frequencies for renal anomalies in FAS are established, it is not clear if routine ultrasound evaluations of the renal system are cost-effective in asymptomatic patients. Certainly, renal evaluations are warranted after any urinary tract infection or when other major malformations are found.

Because growth deficiency is part of FAS, a common medical dilemma remains excluding treatable causes for failure to thrive. There is no standard approach to this problem available in the literature. Children with FAS who are raised in nonabusive and nonneglectful settings and are given appropriate nutrition tend to grow parallel to normal growth curves for length, weight, and head circumference. Therefore, postnatal growth decelerations away from the normal growth curves should not be discounted as simply part of the syndrome. Most frequently, growth deceleration will be due to nutritional insufficiency from poor suck, a lack of interest in feeding, or caregiver neglect. When these problems are excluded and the physical examination does not suggest a specific focus for evaluation, consideration of all the usual reasons for failure to thrive, including problems of infections, absorption, metabolism, tumor, and structure, should be undertaken. Deceleration in the rate of head growth, with or without deceleration in other growth parameters, is very unusual in fetal alcohol syndrome and warrants consideration of brain imaging studies.

Finally, it is important to mention that alcohol exposure can occur in gestations already complicated by chromosomal anomalies or other birth defect syndromes. General syndrome assessment and testing should always be considered in dysmorphic infants who were exposed to alcohol with an "atypical" fetal alcohol syndrome presentation.

Children with fetal alcohol syndrome are reported to have high rates of visual and hearing problems. Visual acuity may be compromised by the short distance from the lens to the retina (small optic globes) or the shape of the lens. Although retinal anomalies may be found, progressive retinal dysfunction has not been reported. Increased frequencies of both conductive and neurosensory hearing problems are found in children with FAS. The frequency of these difficulties and the ages at which they are most likely to become a problem are not fully established. Routine visual screening prior to school and every two years thereafter would appear to be adequate. Similarly, brain stem auditory evoked response (BAER) testing between 6 and 12 months may be of some use in early identification of hearing loss. However, a history of recurrent otitis media or delays in speech should also alert the clinician to the possibility of hearing loss. The efficiency of hearing screening beyond that routinely offered in schools in asymptomatic patients with FAS has not yet established.

Children with FAS frequently have narrow maxillary dental arches and often have Class III occlusion with final mandibular growth. Orthodontic follow-up through middle childhood and transitional dentition may lead to selected dental extractions or other techniques that could prevent more extensive orthodontia or oral surgery.

Severe neurologic problems in FAS are relatively rare. Occasionally, late gestational exposure to alcohol is thought to be a cause of spasticity. Abnormalities in EEGs (electroencephalograms) have been reported in infancy; the rate of seizures is not known, but the possibility of seizures needs to be considered and excluded in patients with histories suggestive of petit mal, absence, or psychomotor seizure forms. Children with FAS appear to go through puberty normally and at the normal age. While there do not appear to be medical problems associated with puberty resulting from prenatal exposure, those young people who are cognitively impaired are at higher risk at this time due to intellectual limitations and impaired judgment. They may also be living in high risk environments.

Finally, it is possible that children with FAS may carry a genetic predilection for alcoholism that can become manifest in adolescence with drug and alcohol experimentation. Early warning and modeling of alcohol avoidance may be helpful, and careful observation of behavior in adolescents is strongly advised.

Behavioral and Social Issues

Research Methodology

In understanding how to meet the needs of individuals with FAS, it is first necessary to describe the behavioral characteristics of affected children as well as the social environment in which many affected children live. Information about affected children is derived mainly from two sources: (1) retrospective and clinical studies of clinically referred children with FAS and fetal alcohol effects, and (2) prospective research studies of children exposed to alcohol in utero due to maternal drinking. In most such prospective research studies, maternal drinking is in the light to moderate range, with only a few women drinking in the heavy range. As a result, most of the children in these prospective studies are not dysmorphic and would not, therefore, qualify for a diagnosis of FAS, although in some cases they may have milder effects that are observable through focused testing or the statistical analysis of group data.

It is well known that these different methodologies often produce different kinds of data and may, if a reader is incautious, suggest different conclusions. (These studies and their outcomes have been reviewed extensively elsewhere and the interested reader is directed to Coles, 1992; Coles and Platzman, 1993; Russell, 1991; and Streissguth, 1986.) In retrospective studies, there is usually much stronger evidence for the effect of a teratogen than in prospective studies, due to the systematic selection biases that occur when children are referred for special education or medical treatment. However, without statistical and experimental controls, it is difficult to discriminate the effects of the teratogen from that of other, associated factors. Despite these limitations, retrospective clinical studies are of great value because the characteristics of the affected individual can be observed much more clearly than among more moderately exposed children. In addition, the characteristics of clinically affected children include those problems that will require intervention and treatment.

In contrast, prospective studies allow some statistical control of confounding variables, as well as the use of contrast groups to control for factors such as social class and race, and also allow examination of factors that can be obscured in clinical studies. However, as described above the sample selected for inclusion in prospective studies is often different from that included in retrospective and clinical studies. The level of prenatal alcohol exposure tends to be less than that found in retrospective studies of identified FAS individuals. This can lead to problems in interpretation of the findings. In interpreting the results of such studies, the problems of overgeneralization and interpretation of multiple comparisons should be considered. For these reasons, in the current review, the type of study from which the information is derived is identified.

Developmental Differences in Clinical Presentation

Children with the full FAS syndrome are distinguished by dysmorphic facial features, growth retardation, and some evidence of damage to the central nervous system (CNS). On average, individuals with the full syndrome are mildly mentally retarded, with IQ scores in the 60s (Streissguth, 1986). However, there is wide variability in presentation, and scores can range from the severely disabled through the average range (85 to 115). Individuals with partial FAS, ARBD, or ARND may have some of the characteristic physical features, while others are absent, or they may have behavioral effects in the absence of physical features. These individuals often have IQs in the "borderline" range (i.e., 70 to 85), and are frequently described in the scientific literature and popular press as having "normal" intelligence. In fact, having intellectual abilities in this range can be very disabling socially and adaptively, particularly if accompanied by the other kinds of problems often found in children growing up in alcoholic families (Brown, 1991; Sher, 1991).

Behavioral deficits have been described by many clinicians. A number of problems have been identified, including (1) attentional problems or hyperactivity (Morse, 1991; Nanson and Hiscock, 1990); (2) academic problems, including specific deficits in mathematics and memory skills (Streissguth et al., 1993); (3) very specific language deficits (Abkarian, 1992); and (4) problems with adaptive functioning that grow more significant with age (Lemoine and Lemoine, 1992; Streissguth and Randels, 1989). Although it is possible to have only one or two behavioral difficulties, in most individuals with a diagnosis of FAS, most of these problems co-occur, which makes an appropriate intervention program hard to implement.

While such patterns are often reported to be characteristic of affected individuals, they are not always seen. Even some dysmorphic children do not show all of these traits (Coles et al., 1994a,b), and in prospectively followed samples of moderately exposed children, few such problems may be seen (N. Day, personal communication, 1994; Greene et al., 1991; Boyd et al., 1991). Although a teratogenic etiology for these patterns is usually assumed, the relationship between specific neurological damage and particular behaviors or patterns of behavioral development has not been well established (see below).

Finally, because of the nature of the developmental process, the behavioral, as well as the physical, manifestations of the teratogenic effect can change over time. Such apparent inconsistencies make diagnosis and treatment difficult and often lead observers to suggest that effects are unrelated to prenatal exposure. However, a better understanding of the meaning of the presentation of behavioral symptoms may also provide a key to their nature.

Newborn and Infancy   Although it would be best to identify affected individuals as early as possible, it is frequently difficult in the newborn period because of the lack of development of specific facial features that are often thought to be more recognizable during the preschool period (Clarren et al., 1987; Egeland et al., submitted for publication; Graham et al., 1988). It has been established (Abel et al., 1993; Coles et al., submitted for publication) that trained observers can identify both the facial features and the behavioral signs associated with prenatal alcohol exposure during this period.

Behavioral patterns characteristic of alcohol-exposed neonates are often those associated with withdrawal from a CNS depressant (Coles et al., 1984, 1985; Nugent et al., 1990; Robe et al., 1981). During the first week of life, infants exposed to sufficiently high amounts of alcohol throughout pregnancy may show excessive arousal, disturbed sleep patterns (Sher et al., 1988), hyperactive reflexes, gastrointestinal symptoms, and other signs of abstinence syndrome. Children who were exposed only during the first part of pregnancy (Coles et al., 1985) or to lower doses (Richardson et al., 1989) may not demonstrate behavioral changes. Behavioral effects, including overarousal and sleep disturbances, may persist over the first month of life (Coles et al., 1987) or longer (Havlicek et al., 1977; Ioffe and Chernick, 1990). Other studies have identified specific behavioral differences in neonates (e.g., habituation deficits relative to controls [Streissguth et al., 1983]; effects on the cry acoustics [Nugent et al., 1990]). (See Coles and Platzman, 1993, for an exhaustive review of effects in infancy and childhood.)

Fewer studies have examined effects in the first two years of life and, often, there have been no effects demonstrated, particularly in samples of children without the full syndrome (e.g., Richardson et al., in press; Streissguth et al., 1980). Growth measures, the metrics of which are more direct and precise than those of behavior, have been found to withstand statistical manipulations sufficiently to allow identification of effects of moderate exposure (Day et al., 1994). Behavior, however, is more slippery to measure and more poorly defined in relation to teratogenic exposure. For that reason, at least, in part only children who are clearly affected (i.e., dysmorphic or growth retarded) or those who are participating in well-controlled prospective studies (Jacobson et al., 1993) have shown effects on global developmental tests during this period.

In contrast, when FAS is identified as clinically significant in infancy and babies are followed medically, there are a number of characteristic problems associated with fetal alcohol exposure, including failure to thrive (often associated with feeding difficulties), delays in development, motor dysfunction, otitis media, and cardiac problems. Behaviorally, infants are often described as having what Greenspan and Wieder (1993) call "regulatory" problems, as well as delays in acquisition of skills. Unfortunately, clinically referred children are often victims of abuse and neglect as well as prenatal exposure and, for that reason, may also suffer from behavioral problems associated with those conditions (e.g., reactive attachment disorder [American Psychiatric Association, 1994] or the behavioral effects of stress), and it can be difficult to discriminate one behavioral effect from another, particularly among individual children in a clinical setting (Zeanah et al., 1993).

Preschool   During the preschool period, usually defined as from $2^1/_2$ to 6 years of age, there are relatively few studies of prospectively followed alcohol-exposed children. Those that have been done are not entirely consistent in their findings across most areas studied, including cognition (Greene et al., 1990; Streissguth et al., 1989), attention (Boyd et al., 1991; Brown et al., 1991; Streissguth et al., 1984), and behavior (Brown et al., 1991; Landesman-Dwyer et al., 1981; Morrow-Tlucak and Ernhart, 1987).

In clinically identified groups, presentation varies, depending on the child's caregiving environment, as well as other factors. However, cognitive deficits are observed frequently, and attention-deficit hyperactivity disorder (ADHD) is often identified (Conry, 1990; Nanson and Hiscock, 1990). Children of this age have been described both as lively, friendly, and socially interested (Streissguth and Giunta, 1988) and also as exhibiting hyperactivity, ADHD, language dysfunction, perceptual problems, and behavioral disturbances (Morse, 1991). Morse et al. (1995) also reported on the frequency of sensory integration problems in a study of a 100 children with FAS and an equal number of controls, finding that parents of children with FAS reported more problems than other parents.

Language Development.   The possibility that there are deficits in language development as a result of prenatal alcohol exposure has been examined, particularly in young children. In children with cognitive deficits, language delays are often noted before other problems and are usually associated with general developmental delay. Of more interest is the possibility that specific language deficits are associated with alcohol exposure. Again, this possibility has been explored both by the examination of children with the diagnosis of FAS and those who clearly have alcohol-related disabilities and by prospective examination of exposed children through identification of maternal drinking prenatally.

In a comprehensive statistical analysis of the first seven years of data from the prospectively followed Seattle sample, Streissguth et al. (1993) concluded that "language disabilities are generally absent from the lists of fetal alcohol effects revealed by these analyses" (p. 198). However, they noted that in clinically referred samples, young children had "good but superficial language skills" that masked the "early neuromotor deficits that foreshadow later school problems" (p. 198). Similarly, a prospective study (Greene et al., 1990) in Cleveland that specifically explored language development in children aged 4 years, 10 months, using both observation and standardized tests, found no evidence of deficits in the exposed groups in comparison with other low-income children.

In a cohort of low-income African-American children in Atlanta, Coles and colleagues also found that language skills were preserved relative to visual or spatial skills and memory (Coles et al., 1991a, 1994a,b). In these studies, language was assessed only as part of a cognitive battery and was confined to measures of vocabulary and fluency, so more subtle deficiencies in language skills may not have been detected.

In another sample, however, Russell et al. (1991) looked at 6 year olds whose middle-class mothers had been identified during gestation as "heavy" drinkers. Among social and moderate drinkers, no significant effects were found on tests of intelligence or on auditory information processing. However, among children of "problem" drinkers (defined from the results of a screening test called Indications of Problem Drinking), scores on the verbal portion of the Weschler Intelligence Scale for Children-Revised (WISC-R), the Token Test (a receptive language measure), and a dichotic listening task were significantly lower than in other groups.

When descriptions of clinical samples of alcohol-affected children's language problems are examined, there is an apparent discrepancy between the child's vocabulary and fluency and the general ability to communicate effectively. Difficulties appear to involve comprehension and social discourse or the pragmatics of speech. These issues were examined by Abkarian (1992), who reviewed the available literature on speech and language disabilities in alcohol-affected children. He concluded that affected children had deficits in the quality of semantics and syntax and in the pragmatic aspects of speech. For instance, although they easily engaged in conversational interactions and understood the need for turn taking, their responses often had little relationship to the initial statements (Hamilton, 1981). In dysmorphic children (Becker et al., 1990), there were indications of articulation deficits associated with structural as well as functional defects.

Abkarian (1992) found that in comparing the experimental and the clinical literature on FAS and alcohol effects, a pattern of communication dysfunction could be identified. This is described as "social but dysfunctional communicative interaction" (p. 232), with individuals being fluid, but superficial, in their speech and having an awareness of the necessity for turn taking without the ability to communicate effectively. Because there are a number of potential reasons for such deficits, the author concludes with a plea for *treatment research* both to describe the nature and extent of any alcohol-related speech and language problems and to identify appropriate methodologies for intervention. Such studies have not yet been done.

School Age   School age covers that time from the beginning of school (usually 6 years of age) until early adolescence (13 years). At this age, clinically referred, affected children are described as unable to sit still in class and pay attention to school work. They are said to find it difficult to deal with multiple sensory inputs, particularly auditory information, and to show significant difficulties in peer relationships (Morse, 1991; Streissguth et al., 1985). Beginning at school age, children have also been reported to "lack remorse," to fail to learn from mistakes, to lack judgment, to be unusually aggressive, and to be unable to maintain friendships (Streissguth, 1992).

Despite the importance of this period of children's academic and intellectual development and socialization, there are few *empirical* studies of the effects of prenatal alcohol exposure during this time. Those controlled research studies that do exist have focused on cognitive performance, academic achievement, and attention or hyperactivity. There is no research-based information available on social and emotional status or other aspects of development in these children.

Cognitive and Academic Performance.   In prospective studies it is at school age that deficits in cognitive performance begin to appear reliably (Coles et al., 1991a; Nanson and Hiscock, 1990), and these have been found even in the absence of physical dysmorphia (Day, personal communication, February 1995; Streissguth et al., 1990).

Streissguth and her colleagues reported that at age 7, cognitive effects, including lower IQ scores on the WISC-R, were associated with heavier drinking during pregnancy in a sample of middle-class, predominantly Caucasian children (Streissguth et al., 1990). In understanding these data, it is important to note that the vast majority of the exposed children were performing in the average range and would not have been identified as showing clinical symptoms. Areas of relative weakness included memory, problem solving, mental flexibility, visual or motor performance, academic skills (measured with the Wide Range Achievement Test [WRAT]), and particularly math skills. These authors also noted that such deficits were more evident under more stressful environmental conditions (e.g., in single-parent families, in large families, and in lower-SES groups). Due to the large sample size, these investigators were able to control most potentially confounding factors.

Similar outcomes were found in a low-SES predominantly African-American sample in Atlanta (Coles et al., 1991a). More impaired performance on the Kaufman-Assessment Battery for Children (K-ABC) was found in children with greater exposure to alcohol. Sequential processing and preacademic skills, particularly precursors to math, were most affected, with language relatively preserved.

Attention. Considerable confusion continues to exist over "attention" as a psychological construct and "attention" as a component of attention-deficit hyperactivity disorder. The latter is defined in the fourth edition of the American Psychiatric Association's Diagnostic and Statistical Manual (DSM-IV) as a constellation of behaviors reported by parents or teachers, and it represents one of the most common problems of childhood. In contrast, attention as the psychological construct is measured by using a variety of tests (e.g., continuous performance [CPT] or vigilance tasks). Children with ADHD do not necessarily exhibit problems in attention, the psychological construct (see Shaywitz et al., 1994, for more extensive discussion of this issue). Although clinicians frequently report disturbances in attention in the offspring of alcoholic women, results from the few systematic studies that address attention in FAS have been difficult to interpret. Thus, Streissguth et al. (1986) found that greater fetal alcohol exposure was associated with poorer test performance on a vigilance task, particularly greater distractibility and more impulsivity. Academic and behavioral deficits consistent with a diagnosis of ADHD were noted in the same children.

A sample from the Atlanta cohort was tested at age 5 years, 10 months (Brown et al., 1991), and a second group of children was tested at 7 1/2 years (Coles et al., 1994a,b), by using two different vigilance paradigms. At 7 1/2 years, a contrast group of children with a confirmed diagnosis of ADHD, who responded therapeutically to stimulant medication, was also tested. At 5 years, 10 months, children whose mothers continued to drink throughout pregnancy showed a relative weakness in sustaining attention across trials but did not demonstrate impulsivity. Hyperactivity and impulsivity were also assessed through standard checklists, videotaped observations, and cognitive measures, and no other ADHD-type effects were noted on any of these measures. At 7 1/2 years, when a more comprehensive assessment of vigilance performance was possible, children with FAS showed better performance on these computerized tasks than did non-alcohol-exposed ("normal") children, while the ADHD-diagnosed children were significantly impaired. Based also on standard checklists and observation of behavior, children with an ADHD diagnosis could be discriminated but children with alcohol exposure were no different from controls.

Similarly, Fried et al. (1992) reported that alcohol exposure (among middle-class, white, social drinkers in Ottawa) resulted in lower levels of impulsivity on a standard CPT task, a finding that is consistent with those in the Atlanta sample but inconsistent with those of Streissguth et al. (1986) and Nanson and Hiscock (1990), who used a group of clinically referred, Native American children in Canada. With a sample of lower-class white and African-American children in Cleveland, Boyd et al. (1991) found no effects of alcohol exposure on attention at age 4 years, 10 months.

There are few studies of older school-aged children who have been exposed to alcohol. In the only prospective study of mild to moderately exposed children *without* dysmorphia who were followed into later childhood, Olson et al. (1992) obtained teacher ratings and academic scores for the Seattle sample at age 11. They found that measures of "binge" drinking (more than five drinks per occasion) during pregnancy were most highly related to later academic difficulties. These children were described by teachers as distractible, restless, and lacking in persistence in contrast to other children in the sample. They were also identified as having problems with processing and reasoning. The authors caution that while similar problems were noted in this cohort of children at 7 years, there were differences in the pattern of deficits from one age to the next. In addition, in this normally functioning cohort, the social problems that were observed at this time were not related to prenatal exposure. Therefore, the impact of prenatal alcohol exposure on school-age children remains to be clarified.

Adolescence   In clinical populations, adolescents with FAS are considered to have significant deficits in intelligence, learning, academic achievement, and—more particularly—in social behavior (LaDue et al., 1989; Spohr et al., 1993). In addition, there are grounds for concern that these youth are at much greater risk for substance abuse than others of this age due to familial exposure and potential effects of their prenatal exposure.

Although the description of school-aged children with FAS is often very negative, adolescents are described in more negative terms still (Dorris, 1989). In a follow-up of German adolescents with FAS and the so-called fetal alcohol effects (FAE), Spohr et al. (1993) identified persistent developmental and psychiatric problems, and described the children's prognosis as "gloomy." Correlations with behavioral outcomes suggested that facial dysmorphia was a strong predictor of persistent pathology. The researchers also noted that in almost all cases, clinically referred children's caregiving environments were "highly disorganized." Lemoine and Lemoine (1992) reported similar outcomes in a 20-year follow-up in France.

Streissguth and colleagues (Streissguth et al., 1991; Streissguth and Randels, 1989) have followed a number of clinically referred individuals, diagnosed as FAS and the so-called fetal alcohol effects, and reported on outcomes in adolescence and young adulthood. Intellectual deficits persisted, as did some dysmorphic features. Puberty was delayed in some males and was associated with weight gain in females. Very poor social outcomes were observed in these affected individuals, with adaptive behavior and social judgment impaired to a greater extent than intellectual functioning. Dysfunctional environments were common (see below). In this sample, as in others, alcohol and other substance abuse was often reported, raising a concern that this group may be at higher risk for such outcomes.

Streissguth and colleagues also have reported on the performance of a large prospectively followed cohort of 14 year olds whose mothers drank moderately during pregnancy. They evaluated attention and short-term memory (Streissguth et al., 1994a), as well as academic performance (Streissguth et al., 1994b), among these clinically normal, middle-class, young people. In examining attention and short-term memory, a number of measures were used, with selection based on the theories of Mirsky (1989). A measure of maternal "binge" drinking—Average Drinks per Occasion, Prepregnancy Recognition—was the best predictor of the child's performance at age 14. Of the 52 outcome measures used, CPT vigilance performance (variable response rate and impulsive responding), Talland letter cancellation (total correct and false alarms), and number of trials on a computerized "stepping stone" maze were most highly related to prenatal exposure.

When two measures of academic ability were evaluated in this same cohort (the Arithmetic Subtest of the WISC-R and the Word Attack Subtest of the Woodcock Reading Mastery Test), there was a significant relationship between academic problems (e.g., "word attack skills" and mathematics problems) and prenatal alcohol exposure in what the authors described as a "dose-dependent" manner. The authors also report a strong correlation between 7-year-old and 14-year-old math performance, particularly among those children showing early deficits whose mothers reported heavy drinking during pregnancy.

Adulthood With the exception of the clinical studies by Streissguth et al. (1991) and Lemoine and Lemoine (1992) cited above, there are no systematic studies of adults with FAS. Thus, there is no information about longevity, sexuality, parenting, vulnerability to disease or mental illness, or other data that would be valuable in planning for these individuals. Anecdotal information suggests that the prognosis is poor and includes a higher risk for substance abuse, criminal behavior, deteriorating mental health, and similar problems. However, it is unwise to generalize from such fragmentary information.

Key Questions for Planning Interventions

For the clinician, as well as the research scientist, there are several important questions that must be answered in order to plan interventions with individuals with FAS, partial FAS, and ARND:

1. *Patterns of development:* Are there discernible developmental patterns among these individuals, so that children can be identified and their development and behavior predicted?

2. *Etiology:* Are the behaviors seen in alcohol-exposed children with alcohol effects the result of prenatal exposure to the teratogen (and thus the result of specific or generalized brain damage); are these behaviors typical of children who have been the victims of abuse and neglect (and thus the result of attachment

disorder, dysfunctional families, and other social problems); or are the behaviors a result of an interaction between brain structure and later experiences?

3. *Specificity:* Are the behavioral deficits reported in alcohol-exposed children specific to FAS and ARND or are they simply secondary to mental retardation or borderline intelligence? If the behaviors seen in children with FAS are no different from the behaviors usually seen in others with mild mental retardation, then no special educational or intervention efforts may be warranted.

Patterns of Development

The first question is whether there are discernible patterns in the development of prenatally exposed children. A review of existing information about the development of these children suggests the following conclusions:

1. *The data base is limited:* Conclusions about individuals with FAS, ARBD, and ARND are based on a relatively few studies. Although there are hundreds of experimental studies (particularly animal models), the information available from well-conducted clinical studies and prospective studies is very limited. The research paradigms that are required to investigate the effects of prenatal exposure arc very difficult to carry out. Working with clinical populations involves difficulties with regard to prenatal exposure to substances of abuse, the clinical populations can be difficult to work with and there are multiple confounding factors. Similarly, the use of longitudinal samples, which provide a rich data base, also has some technical difficulties. It is very labor intensive and financially expensive to carry out such studies. Problems can arise with selective attrition of subjects from the sample and with interpretation of the repeated assessments that are usually done with the sample. Because these samples arc so difficult to identify and follow over time, individuals may be assessed repeatedly with various psychometric instruments, so that the results are subject to possible error due to multiple comparisons. In addition, even when an effect is repeatedly found within the same sample, it is necessary to cross-validate the experiment with a different group to confirm that the outcomes are not a function of the particular sample under study rather than of the "population" of affected individuals in general.

2. *There is a great deal of variability in outcome:* For this reason, it is difficult to generalize about the child with FAS or the alcohol-exposed individual who shows few or less distinct physical signs but is suspected of having behavioral effects (ARND). In some cases, individuals with FAS can be identified during infancy because they show significant deficits early and persistently. More mildly affected individuals have a much more variable developmental course, and it may be difficult to fully discriminate outcomes associated with teratogenic exposure from the effects of other environmental factors in such cases. Finally, many individuals are unaffected by any reasonable criteria.

In addition, because research has been limited, as well as confounded by difficult-to-control environmental factors, firm conclusions about behaviors associated with fetal alcohol exposure are premature.

3. *Early identification is possible in some cases:* Identification is possible in the neonatal period (Abel et al., 1993), particularly in the severely affected child with obvious physical effects and in infants who show behaviors associated with withdrawal.

4. *Effects of prenatal exposure appear to become more significant later in the child's development, perhaps due to the nature of a disorder that may affect behaviors associated with more mature social functioning.*

Effects may be mild during infancy, and many affected children may not meet the criteria for early intervention programs during this time (Coles and Platzman, 1992; Streissguth et al., 1993). This situation may occur for several reasons, including (1) the nature of cognitive and motor development; (2) limitations in measurement of cognitive processes during this time; (3) cumulative effects of the interaction of the biological insult and nonoptimal environments; and (4) the type of neurological damage associated with prenatal alcohol exposure. These possibilities should receive more research attention.

Preschool children with FAS may appear to be friendly and social and to have adequate language skills despite (sometimes) significant cognitive and motor deficits. Among mildly exposed children who have been followed prospectively, language skills appear to be preserved relative to visual or spatial skills, but there are significant (and very specific) deficits in communicative skills in the more affected children who qualify for a clinical diagnosis (Abkarian, 1992).

Cognitive and academic problems are manifest at early school age and appear to involve specific deficits in math skills, some visual or spatial skills, and sequential processing. At this time, in clinical samples, an increase in behavior problems is also reported. These deficits can be identified as early as 5 to 7 years of age with appropriate testing.

Behavioral and social problems appear to worsen with age even in the more mildly affected children. In clinically referred samples, adaptive behavior is not consistent with intellectual ability (Streissguth and Randels, 1989).

Attentional disorders have been widely reported in clinical samples. In empirical studies, there has been very mixed support for this association. Clearly, this is an issue that should receive more research attention, given the potential for misdiagnosis and inappropriate treatment.

In adolescence, affected individuals are reported to have unique neurocognitive and social problems, although most such conclusions have been based on case reports and clinical studies. In addition, alcohol-affected children and adolescents are often identified in minority populations (Coles et al., 1991a; LaDue et al. 1989; Nanson and Hiscock, 1990) and in clinically referred samples (Streissguth et al., 1991), making it difficult to determine whether observed behavior problems result from prenatal alcohol exposure, associated factors such as SES, family dysfunction, and substance abuse, or are secondary effects of mental retardation. Because systematic studies are so rare, there is an even greater need for more empirical research about older children, adolescents, and adults with this disorder than for younger individuals.

Etiology

The second significant question is whether developmental problems seen in alcohol-exposed children should be attributed solely to the effects of the teratogen on neurological functioning, solely to the effects of environmental factors such as social class and dysfunctional families, or to some combination of the two.

At present, there is no easy answer to this question. Although it is logical to assume that outcomes result from interaction between the child's biological status and the caregiving environment, such a statement is too general to provide meaningful guidelines for intervention and treatment.

Neurobiological Markers of Prenatal Alcohol Exposure   Animal studies as well as clinical reports support the belief that prenatal exposure to alcohol affects both the structure and the function of the brain. Support for this view comes from neuropathological studies as well as from more recent reports using newer imaging methods (Clarren, 1986; Mattson et al., 1992; Swayze et al., in press). Together, these reports indicate abnormalities affecting a number of brain regions in many, but not all, affected individuals (see Chapter 4 for a review of this material).

Several investigators have begun to examine the possibility that children with FAS show a similar pattern of deficits to those who have frontal lobe damage (Damasio et al., 1994; Mateer and Williams, 1991; Shallice and Burgess, 1991). Specifically, those persons with FAS show impaired judgment, lability, poor impulse control, and deficits in social and adaptive functioning similar to the kinds of problems seen in patients who have frontal lobe injuries as well as similar learning problems (Santoro and Spiers, 1994).

Most of these data on children with FAS have not yet been published and have been made available only through personal communication (J. Male, July 1994) and presentations at professional meetings (Clarren et al., 1994; Coles et al., 1994a,b; Kodituwakku et al., 1994; Kopera-Frye et al., 1994). However, these few studies present convergent data that strongly suggest that investigation of this area of functioning could provide a useful model for understanding the deficits seen in individuals with alcohol effects.

Environmental Factors Associated with Prenatal Alcohol Exposure   Having briefly described the characteristics often seen in individuals with FAS and

ARND, and having discussed evidence suggesting that neurological damage may account for the associated behavior, it is now necessary to review some environmental factors that must be taken into account in planning intervention and treatment. Because children, including alcohol-affected children, develop within a family and a community, their caregiving environment must be given careful consideration as well. However, although it is widely assumed that the caregiving environments of many individuals with FAS are nonoptimal, the social and environmental factors that may affect their development have not been adequately investigated. Rather, most research efforts have focused on the specific *teratogenic* effects of the prenatal alcohol exposure (see Streissguth et al., 1993) and have treated environmental factors as "confounders." Because such factors may significantly impact alcohol-affected children either independently or interactively, it will be necessary to investigate these issues as well, despite the real difficulty in doing so.

Alcohol abuse and dependence affect the parents' ability to function adequately in many areas (Famularo et al., 1992). Problems often begin during the prenatal period with poor maternal health and inadequate prenatal care (see above) and continue after the birth of the child. For the alcohol-exposed child, as well as all other children, the postnatal rearing environment is of major importance. Alcohol-affected children who remain in the custody of biological mothers who are still abusing alcohol are at risk for failure to thrive and for physical or emotional neglect and abuse (Lemoine and Lemoine, 1992; Streissguth et al., 1985). Even the mother who is attached to the child and well motivated may have inadequate personal resources and social support to enable her to deal with the special needs of the alcohol-affected child (Wilson et al., 1984). This problem occurs, at least in part, because many alcohol abusing or dependent women were themselves reared in dysfunctional families and were themselves the victims of abuse, neglect, and perhaps, prenatal alcohol exposure (Briere and Zaidi, 1989; Cohen and Densen-Gerber, 1982). Because of their own backgrounds, as well as their current life-styles, they may have little to bring to their parenting roles.

For these reasons, an argument can be made that even in the absence of the effects of prenatal alcohol exposure, children might show poorer long-term outcomes due to being reared by addicted parents. There is an extensive literature on the children of alcoholics (Brown, 1991; Earls et al., 1988), and such children are often found to have a higher risk for developmental and behavior problems, probably as a result of unstructured, chaotic, and abusive homes. In addition, research suggests that children of alcoholics are at risk for psychological and emotional problems, including depression, low self-esteem, and learning difficulties (Brown, 1991). However, these findings should be viewed with caution. In such studies, it is often difficult to separate genetic, familial, and environmental factors. In addition, the description of the effects of being the child of an alcoholic varies considerably depending on whether it is from a clinical perspective (Brown, 1991) or from an experimental perspective (Sher, 1991). In experimental studies, effects that are found often are not specific to children of addicted parents but, rather, appear to be the common result of parental dysfunction and psychopathology.

Caregiving Instability: Disruption in the Lives of Alcohol-Affected Individuals
Anecdotal evidence suggests that children with FAS, ARBD, or ARND are more likely to have negative caregiving environments than are typical children or children with other disabilities. The first risk for these children is loss of their biological parents. Some investigators have noted that there is a high mortality rate among alcoholic women who give birth to children with FAS, as well as among women who report using alcohol in pregnancy (Bahna et al., unpublished; Hymbaugh et al., 1995). Spohr et al. (1993) in Germany reported that 11 of 60 mothers of children with a diagnosis of FAS (18.33 percent) had died by a 10-year follow-up. May et al. (1983) found a maternal mortality rate of 23.1 percent at the time of the child's diagnosis in their sample of Native Americans who were assessed between infancy and 17 years (with a mean age of about 6 years). Mena et al. (1986) found a rate of 30 percent (10 of 34) in a Peruvian sample at the time of diagnosis.

Clinical observation also suggests that children with FAS or possible alcohol-related effects often come to the attention of protective service agencies and frequently may enter foster care or be placed for adoption. In 1991, the most recent year for which comprehensive information is available, 429,000 children were in foster care in the United States. This represents an increase of 60 percent since 1986. However, the population of "young children" in foster care (defined as less than 3 or less than 5 years of age, depending on how states kept statistics) increased at a greater rate still. In a General Accounting Office report (U.S. GAO, 1994), three states that accounted for 50 percent of the total number of children in foster care—California, New York, and Pennsylvania—reported an increase of 110 percent in that age group over a five-year period. "Neglect" and "caregiver absence or incapacity" were the primary reasons for the removal of young children from their families in these states (68 percent in 1991). Examination of a random sample of case files at one major location in each state found that 78 percent of young foster children had a least one parent who abused alcohol or other drugs, and prenatal alcohol exposure was explicitly cited in 7.1 percent of these cases.

When clinical studies focus on the caregiving environment of individuals with a diagnosis of FAS, many of these children are reported to have experienced changes of custody and loss of their biological parents. Table 8-1 lists some of these studies and the patterns of caregiving reported in alcohol-exposed children. Because of the way in which data were collected, as well as different laws and customs in different locations, it is sometimes not clear whether children in out-of-home placement are in foster care or with relatives, or whether there have been multiple placements. Institutionalization is rare in the United States at the present

TABLE 8-1 Caregiver Instability Experienced by Alcohol-Affected Children

Study (year)	Location	N	Caregiving Situation (%)				
			At Least One Biological Parent	Foster Care	Adopted	Institutionalized[a]	Multiple Placements[b]
May et al. (1983)	U.S. (southwestern Native American)	128	—	73.3[c]		—	—
Aronson et al. (1985)	Sweden	21	47.6	52.3[c]		—	—
Mena et al. (1986)	Chile	34	53	47% in foster care, with relatives, or in state institutions			—
Streissguth et al. (1991)	U.S. (Native American, Caucasian)	58	22	45	19	7	74
Caruso and ten Bensel (1993)	Minnesota	46	15.2	15.2	8.7	—	—
Steinhausen et al. (1993)	Germany	158	26.6	24.1[c]		25.3	24.1
Egeland et al. (in press)	Alaska	127	—	67		—	—

[a]The percentage of children institutionalized will depend on national and state laws or regulations.
[b]Information about multiple placements is not always available.
[c]The authors did not analyze foster care and adoption separately

time but more common elsewhere. For these reasons, it may be difficult to compare studies. However, despite these differences, it is evident that children affected by prenatal alcohol exposure are at high risk for caregiving instability and loss of family.

In understanding the development and behavior of alcohol-affected children, it is necessary to take these environmental factors into account. Children who have been abused or neglected and who have experienced environmental instability are negatively affected by these experiences. They usually show effects on emotional and behavioral functioning and may have cognitive deficits as well. In designing research and interventions, these environmental factors will have to be considered.

Specificity

Clinical reports suggest that individuals with FAS have behavior problems that are common to most and attributable to alcohol-related brain damage. However, it is not clear that the behaviors reportedly shown by alcohol-affected individuals are different from those shown by other persons who are mentally retarded, have specific learning disabilities, are diagnosed with ADHD, or have been reared in dysfunctional families. Although studies have been done of groups of affected individuals, rarely have these groups been compared to other clinically diagnosed groups to identify factors specific to those who have been exposed to alcohol. For this reason, it is currently unknown whether the behavior problems reported in children and adolescents (Spohr et al., 1993; Streissguth et al., 1991) with FAS are specific to this group or are common to individuals with complex intellectual deficits.

One study compared children with a diagnosis of FAS and the so-called fetal alcohol effects to children of the same age and social status who were diagnosed with ADHD (Coles et al., 1994a,b). Whereas the children were similar in intellectual ability (mean IQ 81.44 versus 82.85), neuropsychological assessment revealed strikingly different patterns of deficits on a number of measures of "attention" (Mirsky, 1989). Although limited in scope, these results suggest that there may be distinct patterns of deficits in alcohol-affected children that can be identified and discriminated from other clinical groups. If it is true that there are specific problems in children with FAS and ARND, it may be possible to design targeted prevention efforts that will help to avoid the more negative outcomes that have been observed.

INTERVENTION AND PREVENTION OF SECONDARY DISABILITIES

Prenatally exposed children are born at biological and social risk, and it is easy to predict that they will eventually show negative consequences. Although

TABLE 8-2 Examples of Interventions to Reduce Prenatal Alcohol Effects

Intervention Point	Intervention Activity	Intended Outcome
Preconception		
Public education	Universal prevention	Improved public awareness of
Substance abuse treatment	Labeling beverages	warnings
Reproductive counseling	Public education	Less drinking in targeted groups
	Targeting specific groups	Reduction of pregnancy in
	Women <45	substance abusers
	Alcoholic women	
	Contraceptive services	
	and counseling	
Prenatal		
Obstetric care	Counseling and education	Fewer pregnant women
Prenatal clinic	about drinking	drinking[a-c]
Substance abuse	Substance abuse treatment	Improved prenatal care
treatment	and case management	Improved pregnancy outcomes
Birth		
Nursery	Neonatal diagnosis,	Improved medical outcome
Obstetrics clinic	identification, and treatment	Reduced future FAS births
	Treatment for mother	Improved mothering
	Periodic developmental	Reduced mortality
	assessment and follow-up	Improved outcome for child
Infancy (0-3 yr)		
Health care clinic	Developmental screening	Improved case finding and
High-risk follow-up	Early intervention services	referral to treatment
(e.g., Child Find)	Medical care	or intervention
Emergency room	Speech therapy	mproved developmental outcome
Protective services	Physical therapy	
	Occupational therapy	
	Emotional, social	
	Foster care placement versus	
	biological parents	
Preschool (3-6 yr)		
Health care clinics	Medical services	Improved health
Pediatricians	Education interventions	Improved parenting
Head Start	Intervention with parents,	
	parenting classes	
School Age (6-12 yr)		
Pediatrician, clinics	Medical services	Improved functioning in home,
School system	Special education services	school, and social settings
Protective services	Specialized service	
Juvenile justice	Counseling; psychotherapy;	
	family therapy	

TABLE 8-2 Continued

Intervention Point	Intervention Activity	Intended Outcome
Adolescence (≥13 yr)		
Mental health system	Symptom-specific treatment	Improved functioning in home,
Juvenile justice	Substance abuse treatment	school, vocational, and
Educational system	Social skills training	social settings
	Vocational training	
	Case management	
	Cognitive rehabilitation	

[a]Olegard et al. (1979).
[b]Rosett and Weiner (1982).
[c]Smith et al. (1987).

in some cases the prenatal exposure may have had permanent effects, it still might be possible to avoid the development of secondary disabilities in these individuals by early identification and appropriate treatment over the life span. Table 8-2 presents an overview of the points in development at which intervention or treatment might be instituted for either parent or child. While these represent points at which interventions could and sometimes do occur, there has been little research done to determine whether there are positive changes in patient outcomes.

It is assumed that many children with FAS or other alcohol effects are receiving medical and therapeutic services of many kinds through private and public programs (e.g., Medicaid and Supplementary Security Income) and educational services through federally mandated Early Intervention Services, Head Start, or Special Education Services when they reach school age. In some states, Child Find and other systems include parental substance abuse or "prenatal exposure" among the indicators of high-risk status, and such children can be routinely referred to tracking programs (see Anderson and Novick, 1992, for an overview of the federal response to the problem of FAS and pregnant women who abuse alcohol). As adults, disabled individuals may be treated in many different public and private systems.

However, although many children and adults affected by alcohol must be receiving services of many kinds, there is no systematically compiled information available describing the number that receive services or the kinds of services received by individuals with FAS or other alcohol-related deficits (Anderson and Novick, 1992). Legislation in 1989 required that state health departments begin annual reporting of the incidence of FAS as part of their responsibilities under the Maternal and Child Health Block Grant Program (U.S. DHHS, 1990). However, it has not always been easy to acquire the necessary information to compile such reports. The Centers for Disease Control and Prevention (CDC) has provided funds to a number of states to facilitate the identification of cases of FAS and to improve surveillance. In many cases, these systems have encountered difficulties due to issues of confidentiality, inaccurate diagnosis in the neonatal period, and the use of different methods of categorization by systems that provide services (see Egeland et al., submitted for publication). For instance, many children with medical conditions related to FAS may not be given the International Classification of Diseases-10 code that specifies fetal alcohol syndrome (i.e., 760.71) but may be identified as showing failure to thrive (783.4), otitis media, mild mental retardation (317.0), developmental delays (319; 783.4), and so on. If the Medicaid, or other medical providers', data systems are accessed, the relationship between these conditions and FAS or ARND may not be evident. Similar problems exist in identifying the number of children who may be receiving Early Intervention or Special Educational Services in the states. Because FAS, ARBD, and ARND are not among the conditions identified as qualifying a child for services, such children will be listed under other, broader categories (e.g., mild mental retardation, behavior disordered, other health impaired). This has negative implications for surveillance, indicated prevention, and treatment.

Medical and Therapeutic Intervention

Children affected by maternal alcohol exposure have intervention needs in numerous areas. They need a primary care physician and may need specialty consultation in neurology, endocrinology, ophthalmology, otolaryngology, and developmental medicine. In order to manage behavior issues they may need psychiatric help with drug management, psychologists to help with behavioral issues and therapists to help the family to come into agreement on how to manage and cope with the alcohol affected individual. Educators, speech and language therapists, occupational therapists, and educational psychologists are almost always needed in helping to develop and monitor individual curricula. Finally the family may need help with social service supports. With adolescent and young adults with FAS there may be the need for birth control, alcohol treatment, and liaison with the criminal justice system.

While the family's physician is often called on to help in organizing the professional care needs of an FAS patient, a primary pediatrician or family physician will often feel ill equipped to handle management which is so complex and requires contact and working relationships with professionals in such disparate disciplines. Therefore it makes intuitive sense that the management of these patients would best be served through development of professional, multidisciplinary teams along a developmental disability model. To date there is no information in the literature describing this model of care with this specific condition and the advantages and drawbacks to this approach.

When the child has been identified through medical or educational screening as needing further services, a comprehensive diagnostic assessment is recommended that should focus on medical, developmental, psychological, educational, social, and adaptive functioning. The particulars of this evaluation will depend on the age and cognitive status of the child. Because of the possibility of fine and gross motor delays, assessment of the infant and preschool child should include physical therapy and occupational therapy assessments. Assessment of speech and language function is also important. While there are almost no data on the effectiveness of such treatment in young children with FAS or ARND, Morse and Weiner (in press) cite two non-U.S. studies (Bierich, 1978; Koranyi and Csilky, 1978) reporting that standard kinds of medical treatment and early intervention services (e.g., occupational therapy) were associated with more positive outcomes.

The efficacy of psychotropic drugs in patients with FAS is not well established. Children are often referred for treatment of ADHD, and methylphenidate is usually the drug first tried for intervention with the symptoms of attention-deficit disorder. The frequency of success with this agent is anecdotally less than in children with ADHD of nonteratogenic cause. When methylphenidate is not successful, other drugs may be helpful, but no specific agents can be recommended at this time.

Educational Interventions for Alcohol-Affected Children

Some, although not all (see below), alcohol-affected children qualify for existing early intervention and special education services. Those who meet the criteria set forth in Public Law 94-142 and Public Law 99-457, which provide for the education of handicapped individuals under 21 years of age, can receive such services. The specific criteria for inclusion in programs are different in different states and even in different jurisdictions within states. In general, children aged 0 to 3 years are served in early intervention programs, and those in kindergarten and above (age 6 to 21) in the school setting. Services for preschool children (3 to 5 years of age) are much less standardized (see Anderson and Novick, 1992; Smith, 1993). Children older than 3 years who are at risk due to social deprivation, as well as other kinds of disabilities, can be served by Head Start programs.

At the present time, there are no empirical studies available of the effects of educational intervention, either generalized (the standard services offered to all qualifying children) or specific (programs specifically designed for those with FAS or ARBD), on alcohol-affected children. A review reveals several types of literature that bear on the issue of educational interventions with this group: (1) articles that review the known characteristics of alcohol-affected children and speculate on the meaning of these characteristics for the educator (Conn-Blowers, 1991; Davis, 1992; Nadel, 1985; Ugent et al., 1986); (2) case studies of children and clinical reports of effective teaching methods like those collected in Kleinfeld and Wescott's (1993) book *Fantastic Antone Succeeds!*; and (3) discussions of programmatic approaches to these problems (e.g., Smith, 1993; Troccoli, 1992; Vincent et al., 1991).

Faced with a lack of published information about teaching methods and the effectiveness of treatment for alcohol-exposed children, Kleinfeld turned to what she called the "wisdom of practice" and collected reports of those experienced in working with FAS (Kleinfeld and Wescott, 1993). Some experienced teachers (Kvigne et al., 1993; Phillpot and Harrison, 1993; Tanner-Halverson, 1993) have developed methods that they find effective in working with alcohol-affected children and, in some cases, have shared these methods with other educators through in-service training and workshops. When these teachers' methods are examined, it is clear that their suggestions are well grounded in an understanding of young children and in practical knowledge about teaching. It is not clear, however, that these methods are of relatively greater value in alcohol-affected children than in other groups.

These suggestions are similar to those mentioned by Vincent et al. (1991) in their discussion of educational methods for children of substance abusers. They mentioned a number of assumptions and techniques that have proved to be useful in the school setting (Cole et al., 1989). These techniques include attitudes toward the child (e.g., the child should be seen as an individual, not a diagnosis), rules about professional relationships (e.g., all professionals involved with the family should meet regularly), and specific classroom techniques (e.g., curricula should be developmentally appropriate and involve experiential learning).

These suggestions, as well as those made by other experienced teachers (e.g., expand a child's verbalization; provide clear, unambiguous rules that are consistently enforced) are all sensible and humane. They are effective methods for use with children in general. However, to determine whether they are more or less effective with children with fetal alcohol effects, evaluation of methods and programs will be required. Such program evaluation should be directed at answering the following questions:

1. *Is the method effective?* Before recommending that a particular strategy or program be used, it first must be tested to see if it improves performance for children in general; for children with FAS or other alcohol effects; and for alcohol-affected children with different characteristics (i.e., age, cognitive status, family structure, clinical history).

2. *What are the effective elements of the program?* If a strategy seems to have potential, it is important to define the specific elements of the program and how each functions. Are all elements equally valuable? Some of the elements to be examined might include specific teaching methods, number of hours in the class, or a particular theoretical underpinning that guides intervention methods.

3. *What aspects of development are affected?* At what aspects of the individual's development is the intervention directed? Are there changes in

outcome associated with various aspects of development—cognitive, social, be-havioral, and so on—as a result of exposure to the methods under study?

4. *Are the effects persistent?* Experience with other intervention programs directed at children with other kinds of developmental disabilities has indicated that effects may not be persistent unless intervention is continued.

Although these questions may seem difficult to answer, similar problems have been addressed in working with other kinds of developmentally affected children. In studying autism, for instance, the parameters necessary to effect positive changes have been established through empirical research (Rogers and Lewis, 1989; Simeonsson et al., 1987). In evaluating the effectiveness of early intervention for low birth weight, high-risk infants, Ramey and colleagues (Bryant and Ramey, 1987) have described the parameters of effective interventions and, therefore, provided recommendations that can be used in designing future pro-grams. Such rigorous evaluations of treatments and interventions can be used as models in designing methods for intervention with children with FAS.

Other Interventions to Improve Outcomes for Affected Individuals

In addition to medical and educational interventions directed at affected individuals, other strategies have been considered to improve outcomes for alco-hol-affected children and adults.

Professional Training and Education of Policymakers

FAS, one of the most common causes of mild and moderate retardation, is often not diagnosed correctly (Little et al., 1990). There may remain a stigma associated with alcohol abuse by women that makes it difficult for professionals to approach them, or the experience of interacting with such families may seem aversive. It may also be true that the training provided to most professionals in this area is not adequate. Research suggests that few professionals working with children have adequate training in identifying and treating the effects of fetal alcohol exposure in children (Good et al., 1990; James Bowman Associates, 1994; Weiner et al., 1988), although programs such as Weiner's that have pro-vided professional education have been successful.

A survey conducted in Washington State in 1994 (James Bowman Associ-ates, 1994) suggested that both the identification of affected individuals and the provision of services could be improved by better training of providers, many of whom, in both public health and social service roles, expressed discomfort in dealing with substance abusers. Problems identified in this area included lack of specific assessment methods and inadequate training of clinicians in making the diagnosis and of those providing education and intervention services. Recom-mendations made as a result of this survey included improved surveillance; enhancement of the availability and accessibility of high-quality diagnostic services; development of a reporting system to monitor FAS, ARBD, and ARND; and improved training of professionals.

Support for Families

Because the child is being reared within a family, whether the biological family or an adoptive or foster family, intervention for the prevention of secondary disabilities in alcohol-affected children must address the needs of the family as well. The way in which this support is provided will depend on the age of the child and the kind of family situation that exists.

In infancy and the preschool period, most early intervention services are carried out in the context of the family. This pattern is generally true in any case, but it is also supported by Public Law 99-457, Part H, which requires that in the provision of treatment to children with developmental disabilities, the family's needs be considered. As a result, much emphasis is currently being placed on family involvement in the process of therapy and intervention. Although there are excellent reasons, both historical and practical, for this emphasis, it may result in difficulties in treating the children of substance abusers if appropriate care is not directed at dealing with such families. Early intervention activities are often based on a middle-class model that assumes more resources, particularly on the part of the child's mother, than may be present. There may also be assumptions made about the efficacy of intervention in infancy (Farran, 1990) and the parents' ability to act as therapists (Seitz and Provence, 1990) that may not be appropriate in families where alcohol abuse is a problem.

In dealing with both families who have produced a child with FAS and those caring for these children in foster or adoptive situations, it is necessary to examine the extent of coping abilities. Most families are stressed by the practical and emotional problems associated with rearing a child with developmental disabilities and the coping abilities of alcoholic families may be especially limited. As a result, such families or such mothers may need more services and support than is usually provided (or available). If the mother is still using alcohol, denial and all the other concomitants of her addiction process will interfere with the child's treatment. If the mother is recovering, the child's diagnosis may be very stressful and may interfere with her recovery process. Guilt over the child's disability will have to be faced and worked through, and plans made for the future. In addition, costs and problems involved in treatment may be overwhelming for a family with limited resources.

Parenting education can be an effective adjunct to other treatments and educational interventions. In women who are addicted to alcohol, childhood traumas often have contributed to current maladjustment. Frequently women have not had the experience of adequate parenting themselves, and their skills as parents are limited. Dysfunctional rules learned in the family of origin can result in a transgenerational cycle of deficient parenting (O'Gorman and Oliver-Diaz, 1987). Parenting education programs with addicted mothers have had demonstrated benefits for both mother and child (Lief, 1981).

Because of the high incidence of abuse and neglect, alcohol-affected children often come into the foster care system or are placed for adoption (e.g., Egeland et al., submitted for publication). Unless well prepared for their care (Bliss et al., 1993) and given adequate systemic support, foster families can be stressed by the special needs of alcohol-affected children who often exhibit the behavioral effects of neglect (attachment disorder), abuse (posttraumatic stress disorder), and poor socialization, as well as the effects of their prenatal exposure. Some adoptive families intentionally choose "special needs" children, but others are as dismayed as biological families to learn that their children are developmentally delayed or otherwise disabled. It may take the family years to realize that the child's impairments will not be outgrown or repaired by their loving care (Dorris, 1989). These families may have to cope with the loss of their hopes for a healthy normal child or their feelings that they can somehow cure the child of this affliction.

Like other parents of handicapped children, families who have adopted children with FAS, ARBD, or ARND are often interested in participating in support groups so that they can share their feelings as well as information about their children. Because adoptive and foster parents often feel a good deal of anger toward the child's biological mother due to her drinking, some prefer separate support groups for foster or adoptive parents and biological parents. Others prefer meeting in joint support groups, finding that in this way the sets of parents are better able to come to terms with each other. Support groups have been formed in a number of states, but their effectiveness has not yet been evaluated.

LIMITATIONS AND BARRIERS TO THE PROVISION OF SERVICES

Although many individuals with FAS and related problems are receiving customary services, not all are eligible for services, and some who are do not come to the attention of social or educational agencies early in life. Some of the problems in providing treatment to alcohol-affected individuals have been identified. The Washington State survey (James Bowman Associates, 1994) noted that there were several reasons why individuals with FAS were not identified. First, FAS is not a recognized diagnostic label in most existing service systems and, therefore, does not establish eligibility for affected individuals. In turn, this lack of diagnostic status prevents access to existing services, particularly for parents who are not able to "negotiate the system." Finally, as discussed above, most alcohol-affected individuals require more than one type of service, and this problem requires that agencies cooperate with each other, which is often very difficult.

Accurate Identification

It has been noted by a number of professionals (e.g., Clarren et al., 1987) that individuals with FAS are sometimes not identified during infancy. It may be very difficult to identify such children. However, it is also true that many health care and educational professionals, particularly those who are working with children beyond early infancy and those in the private sector, are not familiar with the range of effects associated with FAS, ARBD, and ARND, and do not understand the implications of these diagnoses for the child's development. In recent surveys of physicians, nurses, foster parents, and others, respondents have indicated that the majority of their information about the effects of substance abuse in pregnancy came from media reports, many of which are inaccurate (Coles et al., 1991b; Good et al., 1990; Morse et al., 1992; Nanson and Bolaria, 1991).

While most professionals may know that FAS involves facial dysmorphia and the potential for mental retardation, the most frequently described concern is externalizing behavior that is usually attributed to ADHD or hyperactivity (Astley, 1994). Because the research literature (see above) is inconsistent in its findings about the attentional effects of alcohol exposure and because, in the population of abused and neglected children usually referred for assessment, such behaviors may have various etiologies (Zeanah et al., 1993), finding that this is the characteristic most likely to be noted by clinicians is a matter of some concern. Because accurate information about FAS, ARBD, and ARND is not widely known among gatekeeping professionals, many other physical and behavioral problems associated with exposure may be overlooked. In addition, since the full range of problems associated with FAS has not yet been established, there is an understandable lack of experience in dealing with its consequences. A striking example of this problem was presented by Little et al. (1990) who found that of 40 infants whose mothers were identified prenatally as alcoholics, and who had the physical features associated with FAS, none were identified correctly by medical professionals.

Although many providers are willing to serve children with FAS, sometimes it is difficult to identify individuals accurately. At present, there are no universally applied diagnostic criteria or instrument(s) for the diagnosis of FAS, ARBD, and ARND. The Washington State survey (James Bowman Associates, 1994) suggested that the accuracy and efficiency of diagnosis could be improved through more extensive training of a wider range of clinicians and the creation of regional diagnostic centers. The authors also suggested that the confidentiality issues that often interfere with accurate diagnosis be reexamined in order to develop more effective ways of using information while protecting the rights of clients.

Eligibility and Measurement of Development

Another problem is related to the young child's characteristics and the problem of measurement. From infancy through early school age, cognitive deficits are usually "mild" and motor deficits are relatively subtle compared to those usually treated in early intervention programs. Generally, to receive therapeutic services, children must meet state or district criteria, which usually involve standardized testing. Often, to receive services, infants and preschool children must score less than 70 (2 standard deviations [SD] below the mean) on a standardized test in at least one area of functioning (usually cognitive, motor, or language development) or, in some cases 1.5 SD in two areas. Because alcohol-exposed infants may not score in this deficit range during the first year, many do not qualify for services during that time. It might be assumed, given that children do not perform poorly on standardized tests during this time, that they are not really damaged by their prenatal exposure but by other environment factors. However, children with other conditions associated with later deficits (e.g., Down syndrome) may not always score in the deficit range during the first year due to the problem of measurement associated with infant tests. Because the prognosis for children with Down syndrome is well known, however, such children are usually not denied services.

Similar problems can occur when the child is older, as well. Many of the indicators of adult cognitive and emotional functioning are, by definition, missing in infants and preschool children (e.g., language, ability to care for one's self). In currently available data from several sources, alcohol-affected children who will later show mild retardation at school age, score in the low-average range at 12 months and in the borderline range at 24 months (Platzman et al., 1986). These patterns do not result solely from deficits in the validity of test instruments or from poor reliability, but from the nature of the developmental process itself and, probably, from the impact of negative social environments and the particular kinds of brain damage caused by fetal alcohol exposure (see above).

If further research confirms this pattern of declining scores with age, children who need services might not be identified early enough during development to receive preventive treatment but must wait until more severe deficits become manifest. This raises concern, because it is much more difficult to provide useful treatment (see Campbell and Ramey, 1994).

Inconsistency in Follow-Up

Inconsistency in follow-up may be due to many factors. To receive high-quality services, parents of developmentally delayed children must be able to act as advocates with educational and social service systems. When children remain with their biological parents or with relatives, they can be influenced by dysfunction within these families. Because of family problems, which may include the impairments associated with substance abuse, these families can be inconsistent in providing well-baby checkups and immunizations and in following up on medical or educational recommendations (Wilson et al., 1984). Unless severe abuse or neglect brings the child to the attention of authorities, children often will not be noticed until they begin to fail at school or suffer from behavior problems (usually externalizing) that bring them to attention. By this time, usually early school age, it may be difficult to overcome the combined effects of prenatal exposure and lack of educational or medical intervention. When children are in the foster care system, they also may not receive adequate services, for many well-known reasons.

Even when developmental delays are noted, health and educational professionals may not be experienced in dealing with alcohol-abusing parents or with the kind of family dysfunction that often accompanies addiction (Beckwith, 1990). As a result of ineffective interactions with the child's caregivers, treatment recommendations may not be followed. Wilson et al. (1984) identified a number of children with FAS who needed medical and social services. Mothers were noted to have poor psychological adjustment, and half of them were still using alcohol. Because of their own difficulties, mothers were found to be ineffective both in parenting and in their ability to make use of medical or other available services that were needed by their affected children. In another study of low-SES school-aged children prenatally exposed to alcohol, Coles and colleagues (unpublished data) found that although there was a high incidence of medical problems noted in children who could be diagnosed with FAS or possible alcohol-related effects, the use of health care, including checkups, acute care visits, and emergency room visits, was lower in this group than in SES controls.

SUMMARY: INTERVENTION AND TREATMENT

Although the most desirable way of dealing with fetal alcohol syndrome, ARBD, and ARND is through prevention of the birth of an affected child, provisions must be made for affected children when such efforts fail. Efforts to prevent secondary disabilities will involve coordination of several levels of identification, intervention, and treatment in order to maximize the child's postnatal development. Such efforts will also require changes in professional education, application of special educational methods, and changes in some public policy agendas. As such efforts are undertaken, it is important to recognize that although children are affected by prenatal exposure to alcohol, a great deal of neurological development occurs postnatally, and if child care, nutrition, and environment are adequate, it is probable that alcohol-exposed children can make considerable progress. This is particularly true when the insult has not been severe. Among other groups of high-risk children, adequate education and training, together with protection from negative child rearing environments and attention to predictable crises at various developmental stages, can make the difference between achieving a reasonable degree of independence and life satisfaction and more negative outcomes (Campbell and Ramey, 1994).

Negative reports of developmental outcomes for children affected by prenatal alcohol exposure are distressing, particularly when there have been attempts at intervention and prevention over the child's life span. These outcomes have led to the suggestion (LaDue et al., 1989; Spohr et al., 1993) that interventions, including placement in foster care or adoption, do not change the prognosis for children affected by prenatal alcohol exposure. Such negative ideas have affected the way in which children with FAS, ARBD, or ARND are treated by caregivers, health care providers, educators, and social service agencies (Conn-Blowers, 1991; Streissguth, 1992). Clearly, there is a need for better understanding of these issues. However, this understanding will require a number of changes in the approach to this disorder. First, we must provide for a well-organized strategy directed toward investigation of the clinical needs of affected individuals.

RECOMMENDATIONS

The committee concludes that there are no specific programs to treat children with FAS, ARBD, or ARND, and other efforts to prevent secondary disability in these children are insufficient and inadequate. Given the known value of early intervention, however, it is important to identify children with FAS, ARBD, or ARND as early as possible. Thus, in the committee's view, action to bring needed programs and efforts to an acceptable level must proceed on a number of fronts. For example, as pointed out in other chapters, there is a critical need for more consistent diagnostic criteria and better surveillance. Application of these criteria requires the availability of well-trained professionals in social services, education, and health care, as well as those charged with developing policies that impact services for special children. The committee, therefore, recommends the following actions to address these needs:

• Clusters of high-quality diagnostic and treatment services should be available locally and regionally.
• Programs that offer training of professionals and that serve as resource centers for schools and medical clinics should be established.
• Programs serving children with FAS, ARND, or ARBD should meet the special, complex needs of such children, including consideration of the families involved and increased availability of parenting training for caretakers (birth parents, foster parents, and adoptive parents).
• Community outreach programs should be available to establish appropriate lines of communication with clinicians, judges, police, psychologists, teachers, and both birth and adoptive/foster parents.
• Educational materials should be developed for professionals who deal with school-age children to increase their awareness of FAS, ARND, or ARBD as a potential cause of ADHD-like behaviors, including hyperactivity, and to facilitate their referral of such children to other appropriate or needed services.

• Ways should be developed to address the issues of confidentiality that apply to identifying and treating children exposed to alcohol (or other substances) in utero.

• Clinical practice guidelines should be developed for follow-up and treatment of children with FAS, ARND, or ARBD.

A necessary complement to the above actions is an expanded knowledge base. The committee, thus, views further research as essential to providing adequate treatment of children affected by FAS, ARND, and ARBD. The committee recommends additional research in the following areas:

• research to distinguish the role of the postnatal environment in modifying the effects of fetal alcohol exposure, including research on adopted versus nonadopted children with these disorders;

• research on the social and emotional status of school age children affected by FAS, ARND, or ARBD and research on the existence of specific impairments associated with these syndromes, particularly impairments in attention, language, sensory integration, and other behavioral problems;

• further basic research using animal models to examine the underlying neurobiological mechanisms of behavioral and environmental interventions over the life span; and

• evaluation of the effectiveness of educational interventions on children with FAS, ARND, or ARBD, possibly beginning with the examination of educational interventions that look promising in case studies or in studies of children exposed to illicit drugs in utero.

REFERENCES

Abel EL. Fetal Alcohol Syndrome. Oradell, New Jersey: Medical Economics Co., 1990.

Abel EL. An update on incidence in Fetal Alcohol Syndrome: FAS is not an equal opportunity birth defect. Neurotoxicology and Teratology 1995; 17:427-443.

Abel EL, Martier S, Kruger M, Ager J, Sokol RJ. Ratings of fetal alcohol syndrome facial features by medical providers and biomedical scientists. Alcoholism: Clinical and Experimental Research 1993; 17:717-721.

Abkarian GG. Communication effects of prenatal alcohol exposure. Journal of Communication Disorders 1992; 25:221-240.

American Psychiatric Association. Diagnostic and Statistical Manual of Mental Disorders: 4th Edition. Washington, DC: APA, 1994.

Anderson B., Novick E. Fetal Alcohol Syndrome and Pregnant Women Who Abuse Alcohol: An Overview of the Issue and the Federal Response. Washington, DC: U.S. Department of Health and Human Services, 1992.

Aronson M, Kyllerman M, Sabel KG, Sandin B, Olegard R. Children of alcoholic mothers: Developmental, perceptual and behavioural characteristics in children of alcoholic mothers as compared to matched controls. Acta Paediatrica Scandinavica 1985; 74:27-35.

Astley S. Diagnostic Criteria for FAS. Paper presented at CDC Data Collaborative Meeting, 1994.

Aylward GP. The relationship between environmental risk and development outcome. Developmental and Behavioral Pediatrics 1992; 13:222-229.

Barnett R, Schusterman S. Fetal alcohol syndrome: Review of literature and report of cases. Journal of the American Dental Association 1985; 111:591-593.

Bahna DJ, Ammons K, Coles CD. Consequences of alcohol use among women: Mortality rates and specific causes of death. Unpublished manuscript. Available from Human and Behavior Genetics Laboratory, Georgia Mental Health Institute, 1256 Briarcliff Road, N.E., Atlanta, GA, 30306.

Becker M, Warr-Leeper GA, Leeper HA,Jr. Fetal alcohol syndrome: A description of oral motor, articulatory, short-term memory, grammatical, and semantic abilities. Journal of Communication Disorders 1990; 23:97-124.

Beckwith L. Adaptive and Maladaptive Parenting: Implications for Intervention. S. J. Meisels, and J. P. Shonkoff (eds.). Cambridge: Cambridge University Press, 1990:53-77.

Bierich JR. Pranatale schadigungen durch alkohol [Prenatal damage from alcohol]. Der Internist 1978; 19:131-139.

Bliss K, Coles CD, Dugan M, Ellis AM, Wilson G. The Tangled Web: Women, Children and Addiction. Austin, TX: Child Welfare Initiative, 1993.

Bowman [James Bowman Associates]. Washington State Needs Assessment Survey on Fetal Alcohol Syndrome Effects. Seattle, WA: James Bowman Associates, 1994.

Boyd TA, Ernhart CB, Greene TH, Sokol JH, Martier S. Prenatal alcohol exposure and sustained attention in the preschool years. Neurotoxicology and Teratology 1991; 13:49-55.

Briere J, Zaidi LY. Sexual abuse histories and sequelae in female psychiatric emergency room patients. American Journal of Psychiatry 1989; 146:1602-1606.

Brown RT, Coles CD, Smith IE, Platzman KA, Silverstein J, Erickson S et al. Effects of prenatal alcohol exposure at school age. II. Attention and behavior. Neurotoxicology and Teratology 1991; 13:369-376.

Brown S. Adult children of alcoholics: The history of a social movement and its impact on clinical theory and practice. Recent Developments in Alcoholism: Vol. 9 Children of Alcoholics. M. Galanter (ed.). New York: Plenum Press, 1991.

Bryant DM, Ramey CT. An Analysis of the Effectiveness of Early Intervention Programs for Environmentally At-Risk Children. The Effectiveness of Early Intervention for At-Risk and Handicapped Children. M.J. Guralnick and F.C. Bennett (eds.). Orlando, FL: Academic Press, 1987.

Campbell FA, Ramey CT. Effects of early intervention on intellectual and academic achievement: A follow-up study of children from low-income families. Child Development 1994; 65:684-698.

Caruso K, ten Bensel R. Fetal alcohol syndrome and fetal alcohol effects. Minnesota Medicine 1993; 76:25-29.

Chappel JN. Attitudinal barriers to physician involvement with drug abusers. Journal of the American Medical Association 1973; 224:1011-1013.

Church MW, Gerkin KP. Hearing disorders in children with fetal alcohol syndrome: Findings from case reports. Pediatrics 1988; 82:147-154.

Clarren SK. Neuropathology in Fetal Alcohol Syndrome. Alcohol and Brain Development. J. R. West (ed.) New York: Oxford University Press, 1986:158-166.

Clarren SB, Clarren SK, Astley SJ, Shurtleff H, Unis A, Weinberger E. A Neurodevelopmental, Psychoeducational Profile of Children with Fetal Alcohol Syndrome. Paper presented at Symposium, Research Society on Alcoholism Annual Meeting 1994.

Clarren SK, Sampson PD, Larsen J, Donnell DJ, Barr HM, Bookstein FL et al. Facial effects of fetal alcohol exposure: Assessment by photographs and morphometric analysis. American Journal of Medical Genetics 1987; 26:651-666.

Cohen FS, Densen-Gerber J. A study of the relationship between child abuse and drug addiction in 178 patients: Preliminary results. Child Abuse and Neglect 1982; 6:383-387.

Cole C, Ferrara V, Johnson C, Jones M, Schoenbaum M, Tyler R, et al. Today's challenge: Teaching strategies for working with young children pre-natally exposed to drugs/alcohol. Los Angeles, CA: Los Angeles Unified School District, 1989.

Coles CD. Prenatal Alcohol and Human Development. Development of the Central Nervous System: Effects of Alcohol and Opiates. M. Miller (ed.). New York: Wiley-Liss, 1992.

Coles CD, Brown RT, Raskind-Hood CL, Platzman KA, Smith IE, Falek A. A comparative study of neurocognitive functioning in fetal alcohol (FAS) and attention deficit, hyperactivity disorder (ADHD). Paper presented at Symposium, Research Society on Alcoholism Annual Meeting 1994a.

Coles CD, Brown RT, Smith IE, Platzman KA, Erickson S, Falek A. Effects of prenatal alcohol exposure at 6 years: I. Physical and cognitive development. Neurotoxicology 1991a; 13:1-11.

Coles CD, Krebs K, Smith IE, Morse B, Weiner L. Identification and treatment of fetal alcohol syndrome: Pediatricians' perspectives (Abs.). Alcoholism: Clinical and Experimental Research 1991b; 15:369.

Coles CD, Platzman KA. Fetal alcohol effects in preschool children: Research, prevention, and intervention. OSAP Technical Manual, Drug Exposed Children, Ages 2-5: Identifying their needs and planning for early intervention. Rockville, MD: Office of Substance Abuse Prevention, 1992.

Coles CD, Platzman KA. Behavioral development in children prenatally exposed to drugs and alcohol. International Journal of the Addictions 1993; 28:1393-1433.

Coles CD, Raskind-Hood CL, Brown RT, Silverstein JD. A comparison of information processing in children with fetal alcohol effects and attention deficit disorder. Poster presented at the Research Society on Alcoholism Annual Meeting, 1994b.

Coles CD, Smith IE, Fernhoff PM, Platzman KA, Raskind-Hood CL, Brown RT et al. Consistency of effects of prenatal alcohol exposure: Prediction from the neonatal period. Submitted for publication.

Coles CD, Smith ID, Fernhoff PM, Falek A. Neonatal ethanol withdrawal: Characteristics in clinically normal, nondysmorphic neonates. Journal of Pediatrics 1984; 105:445-451.

Coles CD, Smith I, Fernhoff PM, Falek A. Neonatal neurobehavioral characteristics as correlates of maternal alcohol use during gestation. Alcoholism: Clinical and Experimental Research 1985; 9:454-460.

Coles CD, Smith IE, Lancaster JS, Falek A. Persistence over the first month of neurobehavioral alterations in infants exposed to alcohol prenatally. Infant Behavior and Development 1987; 10:23-37.

Conn-Blowers EA. Nurturing and educating children prenatally exposed to alcohol: The role of the counsellor. International Journal for the Advancement of Counselling 1991; 14:91-103.

Conry J. Neuropsychological deficits in fetal alcohol syndrome and fetal alcohol effects. Alcoholism: Clinical and Experimental Research 1990; 14:650-655.

Damasio H, Grabowski T, Frank R, Galaburda AM, Damasio AR. The return of Phineas Gage: Clues about the brain from the skull of a famous patient. Science 1994; 264:1102-1105.

Davis D. The FAS/FAE child in the classroom. The Iceberg: An Educational Letter on FAS/FAE. 1992.

Day NL, Richardson GA, Geva D, Robles N. Alcohol, marijuana, and tobacco: Effects of prenatal exposure on offspring growth and morphology at age six. Alcoholism: Clinical and Experimental Research 1994; 18:786-794.

Dorris M. The Broken Cord. New York: Harper & Row, 1989.

Earls F, Reich W, Jung KG, Cloninger R. Psychopathology in children of alcoholic and antisocial parents. Alcoholism: Clinical and Experimental Research 1988; 12:481-487.

Egeland GM, Perham-Hester KA, Gessner BD, Ingle D, Berner J, Middaugh JP. Fetal alcohol syndrome in Alaska. Submitted for publication.

Famularo R, Kinscherff R, Fenton T. Parental substance abuse and the nature of child maltreatment. Child Abuse and Neglect 1992; 16:475-483.

Farran DC. Effects of Intervention with Disadvantaged and Disabled Children: A Decade Review. Handbook of Early Childhood Intervention. S. J. Meisels and J. P. Shonkoff (eds.). Cambridge: Cambridge University Press, 1990.

Fried PA, Watkinson B, Gray R. A follow-up study of attentional behavior in 6-year-old children exposed prenatally to marihuana, cigarettes, and alcohol. Neurotoxicology and Teratology (United States) 1992; 14:299-311.

Good LN, Strickland KE, Coles CD. Knowledge and attitudes of public and professionals about substance abuse in pregnancy. Presented at the Committee on Problems of Drug Dependency Annual Meeting, Richmond, VA, June 10-14, 1990.

Graham JM, Hanson JW, Darby BL, Barr HM, Streissguth AP. Independent dysmorphology evaluations at birth and 4 years of age for children exposed to varying amounts of alcohol in utero. Pediatrics 1988; 81:772-778.

Greene T, Ernhart CB, Martier S, Sokol RJ, Ager J. Prenatal alcohol exposure and language development. Alcoholism: Clinical and Experimental Research 1990; 14:937-945.

Greene T, Ernhardt CB, Ager H, Sokol R, Martier S, Boyd T. Prenatal alcohol exposure and cognitive development in the preschool years. Neurotoxicology and Teratology 1991; 13:57-68.

Greenspan SI, Wieder S. Regulatory disorders. Handbook of Infant Mental Health. C.H. Zeanah (ed.). New York: Guilford Press, 1993.

Hamilton M. Linguistic abilities of children with fetal alcohol syndrome. Unpublished masters thesis, University of Washington, Seattle 1981.

Hannigan JH, Berman RF, Zajac CS. Environmental enrichment and the behavioral effects of prenatal exposure to alcohol in rats. Neurotoxicology and Teratology 1993; 15:261-266.

Havlicek V, Childiaeva R, Chernick V. EEG frequency spectrum characteristics of sleep states in infants of alcoholic mothers. Neuropadiatrie 1977; 8:360-373.

Hymbaugh KJ, May PA, Aase JM. Observations on ARBD and maternal age and birth order in a large case series of American Indians. Paper presented for symposium on "Increased Vulnerability to the Effects of Fetal Alcohol Exposure in Infants Born to Older Mothers." J. Jacobson, Chair. Research Society on Alcoholism Annual Meeting, Steamboat Springs, CO, June 18, 1995.

Ioffe S, Chernick V. Prediction of subsequent motor and mental retardation in newborn infants exposed to alcohol in utero by computerized EEG analysis. Neuropediatrics 1990; 21:11-17.

Jacobson JL, Jacobson SW, Sokol RJ, Martier SS, Ager JW, Kaplan-Estrin MG. Teratogenic effects of alcohol on infant development. Alcoholism: Clinical and Experimental Research 1993; 17: 174-183.

Kleinfeld J, Wescott S. Fantastic Antone Succeeds!: Experiences in Educating Children with Fetal Alcohol Syndrome. Fairbanks, AK: University of Alaska Press, 1993.

Kodituwakku PW, Handmaker NS, Weathersby EK, Cutler SK, Handmaker SD. Impaired goal management in working memory in FAS/FAE. Poster presented at the Research Society on Alcoholism Annual Meeting 1994.

Kopera-Frye K, Dehaene S, Streissguth AP. Cognitive deficits in number processing evident in alcohol-affected young adults. Poster presented at the Research Society on Alcoholism Annual Meeting 1994.

Koranyi G, Csilky E. Az embryopathia gyermekkorban eszleheto tuneteirol [Signs of alcohol embryopathy apparent in childhood]. Orvosi Hetilap 1978; 119:2923-2929.

Kvigne V, Struck H, Engelhart E, West T. Appendix I: Education Techniques for Children with FAS/FAE. Fantastic Antone Succeeds: Experiences in Educating Children with Fetal Alcohol Syndrome. J. Kleinfeld and S. Wescott (eds.). Fairbanks, AK: University of Alaska Press, 1993.

LaDue RA, Streissguth AP, Randels SP. Clinical considerations pertaining to adolescents and adults with fetal alcohol syndrome. In: Sonderegger T. (ed.). Perinatal Substance Abuse: Research Findings and Clinical Implications. Baltimore: Johns Hopkins University Press, 1989.

Landesman-Dwyer S, Ragozin AS. Behavioral correlates of prenatal alcohol exposure: A four-year follow-up study. Neurobehavioral Toxicology 1981; 3:187-193.

Lemoine P, Lemoine H. Avenir des enfants de meres alcoliques (etude de 105 das retrouves a l'age adulte) et qelques constatations d'interet prophalactique. Annales de Pediatrie (Paris) 1992; 39:226-235.

Lief N. Parenting and Child Services for Drug Dependent Women. Treatment Services for Drug Dependent Women. G. M. Breschner, B. G. Reid, and J. Mondanaro (eds.) Washington, DC: U.S. Government Printing Office, 1981:455-498.

Little BB, Snell LM, Rosenfeld CR, Gilstrap LCI, Gant NF. Failure to recognize fetal alcohol syndrome in newborn infants. American Journal of Disease in Children 1990; 144:1142-1146.

Mateer CA, Williams D. Effects of frontal lobe injury in childhood. Development Neuropsychology 1991; 7:359-376.

Mattson SN, Riley EP, Jernigan TL, Ehlers CL, Delis DC, Jones KL et al. Fetal alcohol syndrome: A case report of neuropsychological, MRI and EEG assessment of two children. Alcoholism: Clinical and Experimental Research 1992; 16:1001-1003.

May PA, Hymbaugh KJ, Aase JM, Samet JM. Epidemiology of fetal alcohol syndrome among American Indians of the Southwest. Social Biology 1983; 30:374-387.

Meisels SJ, Shonkoff JP. Handbook of Early Childhood Intervention. Cambridge: Cambridge University Press, 1990.

Mena M, Casaneuva V, Fernandez E, Carrasco V, Perez H. Fetal Alcohol Syndrome at schools for mentally handicapped children in Concepcion, Chile. Bulletin of the Pan American Health Organization 1986; 20:157-169.

Mirsky AF. The neuropsychology of attention: Elements of a complex behavior. Integrating Theory and Practice in Clinical Neuropsychology. E. Peregman (ed.). Hillsdale, NJ: Lawrence Erlbaum Associates, 1989.

Morrow-Tlucak M, Ernhart CB. Maternal perinatal substance use and behavior at age 3 years (Abs.). Alcoholism: Clinical and Experimental Research 1987; 11:213.

Morse BA. Fetal alcohol syndrome in the developing child. Paper presented at the Fetal Alcohol Syndrome and Other Congenital Alcohol Disorders: A National Conference on Surveillance and Prevention, Centers for Disease Control, Atlanta, GA. 1991.

Morse BA, Weiner L. Rehabilitation approaches for FAS. Alcohol, Pregnancy, and the Developing Child. H. Spohr and H. Steinhausen (eds.). In press.

Morse BA, Idelson RK, Sachs WH, Weiner L, Kaplan LC. Pediatricians' perspectives on Fetal Alcohol Syndrome. Journal of Substance Abuse 1992; 4:187-195.

Morse BA, Miller AL, Cermak SA. Sensory processing in children with fetal alcohol syndrome (abstract). Alcoholism: Clinical and Experimental Research 1995; 19:101a

Nadel M. Offspring with fetal alcohol effects: Identification and intervention. Alcoholism Treatment Quarterly 1985; 2:105-116.

Nanson JL, Bolaria MA. Physician's awareness of fetal alcohol syndrome: A survey of pediatricians and general practitioners (Abs.). Alcoholism: Clinical and Experimental Research 1991; 15:367.

Nanson JL, Hiscock M. Attention deficits in children exposed to alcohol prenatally. Alcoholism: Clinical and Experimental Research 1990; 14:656-661.

Nugent JK, Lester BM, Greene S. Maternal alcohol use during pregnancy and acoustic cry analysis. Presented at the 7th International Conference on Infant Studies, Montreal, Canada. 1990.

O'Gorman P, Oliver-Diaz P. Breaking the cycle of addiction: A parent's guide to healthy kids. Pompano Beach, FL: Health Communications, 1987.

Olegard R, Sabvel KG, Aronsson J, Sandin B, Johnsson PR, Carlsson C et al. Effects on the child of alcohol abuse during pregnancy: Retrospective and prospective studies. Acta Paediatrica Scandinavica 1979; 275 (Supplement):112-121.

Olson HC, Sampson PD, Barr H, Streissguth AP, Bookstein FL. Prenatal exposure to alcohol and school problems in late childhood: A longitudinal perspective study. Developmental Psychopathology 1992; 4:341-359.

Phillpot B, Harrison N. A one-room schoolhouse for children with FAS/FAE. Fantastic Antone Succeeds: Experiences in Educating Children with Fetal Alcohol Syndrome. J. Kleinfeld and S. Wescott (eds.). Fairbanks, AK: University of Alaska Press, 1993.

Platzman KA, Coles CD, Rubin CP, Smith IE. Developmental profiles of infants with fetal alcohol syndrome and fetal alcohol effects. Presented at the Southeastern Psychological Association Annual Meeting, Orlando, FL. 1986.

Richardson GA, Day NL, Taylor PM. The effect of prenatal alcohol, marijuana, and tobacco exposure on neonatal behavior. Infant Behavior and Development 1989; 12:199-209.

Richardson GA, Day NL, Goldschmidt L. Prenatal alcohol, marijuana, and tobacco use: Infant mental and motor development. Neurotoxicology and Teratology. In press.

Robe LB, Gromisch DS, Isoub S. Symptoms of neonatal ethanol withdrawal. Currents in Alcoholism 1981; 8:485-493.

Robinson LH, Podnos B. Resistance of psychiatrists in treatment of alcoholism. Journal of Nervous and Mental Disorders 1966; 143:220-225.

Rogers S, Lewis H. An effective day treatment model for young children with pervasive developmental disorders. Journal of American Academy of Child and Adolescent Psychiatry 1989; 32:1274-1282.

Rosett HL, Weiner L. Prevention of fetal alcohol effects. Pediatrics 1982; 69:813-816.

Russell M. Clinical implications of recent research on the fetal alcohol syndrome. Bulletin of the New York Academy of Medicine 1991; 67:207-222.

Russell M, Czarnecki DM, Cowan R, McPherson E, Mudar PJ. Measures of maternal alcohol use as predictors of development in early childhood. Alcoholism: Clinical and Experimental Research 1991; 15:991-1000.

Santoro J, Spiers M. Social cognitive factors in brain injury-associated personality change. Brain Injury 1994; 8:265-276.

Seitz V, Provence S. Caregiver-focused models of early intervention. Handbook of Early Childhood Intervention. New York: Cambridge University Press, 1990.

Shallice T, Burgess PW. Deficits in strategy application following frontal lobe damage in man. Brain 1991; 114:727-741.

Shaywitz SE, Fletcher JM, Shaywitz BA. Issues in the definition and classification of attention deficit disorder. Topics in Language Disorders 1994; 14:1-25.

Sher KJ. Psychological characteristics of children of alcoholics: Overview of research methods and findings. Recent Developments in Alcoholism V. 9: Children of Alcoholics. New York: Plenum Press, 1991.

Sher MS, Richardson GA, Coble PA, Day NL, Stoffer DS. The effects of prenatal alcohol and marijuana exposure: Disturbances in neonatal sleep cycling and arousal. Pediatric Research 1988; 24:101-105.

Simeonsson RJ, Olley JG, Rosenthal SL. Early intervention for children with Autism. The Effectiveness of Early Intervention for At-Risk and Handicapped Children. M.J. Guralnick and F.C. Bennett (eds.). Orlando, FL: Academic Press, 1987.

Smith GH. Intervention strategies for children vulnerable for school failure due to exposure to drugs and alcohol. International Journal of the Addictions 1993; 28:1435-1470.

Smith IE, Coles CD. Multilevel intervention for prevention of fetal alcohol syndrome and effects of prenatal alcohol exposure. Recent Developments in Alcoholism, Vol. 9. M. Galanter (ed.). New York: Plenum, 1991.

Smith IE, Lancaster JS, Moss-Wells S, Coles CD, Falek A. Identifying high-risk pregnant drinkers: Biological and behavioral correlates of continuous heavy drinking during pregnancy. Journal of Studies on Alcohol 1987; 48:304-309.

Spohr HL, Willms J, Steinhausen JC. Prenatal alcohol exposure and long-term developmental consequences. Lancet 1993; 341:907-910.

Steinhausen HC, Willms J, Spohr HL. Long-term psychopathology and cognitive outcome of children with fetal alcohol syndrome. Journal of the American Academy of Child and Adolescent Psychiatry 1993; 32:990-1006.

Streissguth AP. The behavioral teratology of alcohol: Performance, behavioral and intellectual deficits in prenatally exposed children. Alcohol and Brain Development. J. West (ed.). New York: Oxford University Press, 1986.

Streissguth AP. Fetal alcohol syndrome and fetal alcohol effects: A clinical perspective of later developmental consequences. Maternal Substance Abuse and the Developing Nervous System. I. S. Sagon and T. A. Slotkin (eds.). San Diego, CA: Academic Press, Inc., 1992.

Streissguth AP, Randels SP. Long term effects of fetal alcohol syndrome. Alcohol and Child/Family Health. G. Robinson (ed.). Vancouver, Canada: University of British Columbia Press, 1989.

Streissguth AP, Giunta CT. Mental health and health needs of infants and preschool children with Fetal Alcohol Syndrome. International Journal of Family Psychiatry 1988; 9:29-47.

Streissguth AP, Aase JM, Clarren SK, Randels SP, LaDue RA, Smith DF. Fetal alcohol syndrome in adolescents and adults. Journal of the American Medical Association 1991; 265:1961-1967.

Streissguth AP, Barr HM, Sampson PD, Parrish-Johnson JC, Kirchner GL, Martin DC. Attention, distraction and reaction time at age 7 years and prenatal alcohol exposure. Neurobehavioral Toxicology and Teratology 1986; 8:717-725.

Streissguth AP, Barr HM, Olson HC, Sampson PD, Bookstein FL, Burgess DM. Drinking during pregnancy decreases word attack and arithmetic scores on standardized tests: Adolescent data from a population-based prospective study. Alcoholism: Clinical and Experimental Research 1994a; 18:248-254.

Streissguth AP, Barr HM, Martin DC, Harman CS. Effects of maternal alcohol, nicotine and caffeine use during pregnancy on infant and motor development at eight months. Alcoholism: Clinical and Experimental Research 1980; 4:152-164.

Streissguth AP, Barr HM, Sampson PD, Darby BL, Martin DC. IQ at age 4 in relation to maternal alcohol use and smoking during pregnancy. Developmental Psychology 1989; 25:3-11.

Streissguth AP, Barr HM, Martin DC. Maternal alcohol use and neonatal habituation assessed with the Brazelton Scale. Child Development 1983; 54:1109-1181.

Streissguth AP, Barr HM, Sampson PD. Moderate prenatal alcohol exposure: Effects on child IQ and learning problems at age 7.5 years. Alcoholism: Clinical and Experimental Research 1990; 14:662-669.

Streissguth SP, Bookstein FL, Sampson PC, Barr HM. The Enduring Effects of Prenatal Alcohol Exposure on Child Development: Birth Through Seven Years, a Partial Least Squares Solution. Ann Arbor, MI: University of Michigan Press, 1993.

Streissguth AP, Clarren SK, Jones KL. Natural history of the fetal alcohol syndrome: A 10-year follow-up of eleven patients. Lancet 1985; 2:85-92.

Streissguth AP, Martin DC, Barr HM, Sandman BM, Kirchner GL, Darby BL. Intrauterine alcohol and nicotine exposure: Attention and reaction time in 4-year-old children. Developmental Psychology 1984; 20:533-541.

Streissguth AP, Sampson PD, Olson HC, Bookstein FL, Barr HM, Scott M et al. Maternal drinking during pregnancy: Attention and short-term memory in 14-year-old offspring—A longitudinal prospective study. Alcoholism: Clinical and Experimental Research 1994b; 18:202-218.

Stromland K. Eyeground malformations in the fetal alcohol syndrome. Neuropediatrics 1981; 12:97-98.

Swayze VW, Johnson VP, Hanson JW, Piven J, Sato Y, Andreasen NC. Magnetic resonance imaging of midline brain anomalies in fetal alcohol syndrome. In press.

Tanner-Halverson P. Snagging the kite string. Fantastic Antone Succeeds: Experiences in Educating Children with Fetal Alcohol Syndrome. J. Kleinfeld and S. Wescott (eds.). Fairbanks, AK: University of Alaska Press, 1993.

Troccoli KB. Fetal Alcohol Syndrome: The impact on children's ability to learn. National Health/Education Consortium—Occasional Paper #10. 1992.

Ugent WD, Graff MH, Ugent AS. Fetal Alcohol Syndrome: A problem that school psychologists can help recognize, treat and prevent. School Psychology International 1986; 7:55-60.

U.S. Department of Health and Human Services, Public Health Service, Office of Disease Prevention and Health Promotion (ODPHP). Healthy People 2000: National Health Promotion and Disease Prevention Objectives. Conference Edition. U.S. DHHS: Washington, D.C., September 1990.

U.S. General Accounting Office, Report to the Chairman, Subcommittee on Human Resources, Committee on Ways and Means, House of Representatives. Foster Care: Parental Drug Abuse has Alarming Impact on Young Children. Washington, DC: U.S. General Accounting Office, 1994.

Vincent LH, Poulsen MK, Cole CK, Woodruff G, Griffith DR. Born substance exposed, educationally vulnerable. Reston, VA: Council for Exceptional Children, 1991.

Weinberg J, Kim CK, Ju W. Early handling can attenuate adverse effects of fetal ethanol exposure. Alcohol; in press.

Weiner L, McCarty D, Potter DA. A successful in-service training program for health care professionals. Substance Abuse 1988; 9:20-28.

Wilson PJ, Scott RV, Briggs FH, Ince SE, Quinton BS, Headings VE. Characteristics of parental response to fetal alcohol syndrome. Strategies in Genetic Counseling: Clinical Investigation Studies. B. S. Fine and N. W. Paul (eds.). White Plains, NY: March of Dimes Birth Defects Foundation, 1984.

Zeanah CH, Mammen OK, Lieberman AF. Disorders of attachment. Handbook of Infant Mental Health. C.H. Zeanah (ed.). New York: Guilford Press, 1993.

9
Integration and Coordination: A Concluding Comment and Recommendation

There is no single, organized discipline within medicine that can, at this time, logically be held responsible or accountable for the development of a comprehensive approach to preventing and treating fetal alcohol syndrome (FAS), alcohol-related neurodevelopmental disorder (ARND), or alcohol-related birth defects (ARBD). Nor is there a single discipline in the broader arena of health and health care appropriate for this role. The problem is obvious. Primary care health care providers are frequently presented with the opportunity to detect substance abuse and make referrals for treatment. Psychiatrists and other mental health care workers also are responsible for recognizing and treating substance abuse and dependence. Obstetricians and family physicians are concerned principally with the prevention and management of teratogenic exposures, while pediatricians and family physicians manage birth defects in infants. Because the disorders pose health and developmental problems over the life span, they have been variably managed after the newborn period by pediatric subspecialists such as clinical geneticists, developmentalists, child neurologists, and others. No group has yet shown any interest in the management of FAS, ARBD, or ARND patients as adults. Families affected by FAS frequently require the services of specialists in substance abuse, developmental disabilities, and education. Therefore, these disorders lie within the purview of many groups but are clearly not the full responsibility of any one. All groups will accept, or have accepted, an interest in handling an appropriate piece of the problem, but no one is in a position to lead and coordinate. Hence, there is no group to which government can look for leadership, and no group is focused on advocacy or comprehensive education about the disorders. Attention to FAS, ARBD, and ARND, then, is structurally marginalized, and like any problem that falls between organized disciplines, progress is unavoidably hampered. Both FAS research and service delivery suffers.

Such structural marginalization is also evident in government, where it is difficult to find a government system that is positioned to address these disorders in a comprehensive manner. The National Institute on Alcohol Abuse and Alcoholism (NIAAA) has lead responsibility for research on alcohol and historically has played the major role in FAS research. The Centers for Disease Control and Prevention recently has expanded its FAS activities beyond surveillance into prevention. The Substance Abuse and Mental Health Services Agency (SAMHSA) funds prevention and treatment demonstration projects for substance-abusing pregnant women, including women at risk for having a child with FAS. The Health Services and Resources Administration co-funds some of the SAMHSA programs and sponsors maternal and child health projects. The Indian Health Service provides services to some populations at risk for FAS and other alcohol-related problems. No agency has assumed responsibility for research on interventions with people affected by FAS, ARBD, or ARND. No agency has responsibility for coordinating the many services needed by families affected by FAS and related disorders.

It is often difficult to achieve meaningful cooperation among government research and services agencies for a given problem. Such cooperation, however, can be facilitated by willingness of individual personnel to move beyond the structural barriers of government bureaucracies. In most state governments, agencies responsible for child neglect and abuse, foster and adoptive care, health, education, criminal justice, and alcohol treatment are distinct entities. Yet, interagency coordination of personnel and budgets is needed for state governments to help patients and their families affected by FAS, ARND, or ARBD, without involving the criminal justice and social service systems that are focused on child abuse. At the federal level, there is similarly no single agency responsible for all the programs or research needed.

It is clear that neither governmental structures nor the organization of modern medicine and health care can be redesigned. Thus, the challenge is to improve communication and cooperation among health, education, and social services disciplines and government agencies. The committee believes that such cooperation may best be addressed by the recommendations made to increase professional education about FAS and its related disorders, and to establish clinical practice guidelines for the management of patients and their families (see Chapters 7 and 8). Further, the committee believes that any possible coordination at a state level will depend first on leadership shown by federal agencies to communicate with each other and to coordinate programmatic goals and objectives.

• Therefore, the committee recommends that an interagency task force, or other entity comprised of representatives from the relevant federal research, surveillance, and services agencies, be established to coordinate national efforts in FAS, ARND, and ARBD.

Lead responsibility for heading this task force should be assigned to NIAAA, because it is experienced at encouraging research and at incorporating research methodologies into all activities and has had the longest history in addressing FAS. However, all member agencies should be willing and able to translate research findings into service delivery and policy development activities and be expected to contribute to and be consulted with about achieving the overall goals of preventing FAS.

It is suggested that one of the top priorities of such a coordinating body should be to forge interagency cooperation in the adoption of a common terminology and set of definitions related to these disorders, such as proposed in this report, and the design and implementation of national surveys to estimate the true prevalence of FAS, ARND, and ARBD. At the same time, prevention and treatment of secondary disabilities associated with FAS, ARND, and ARBD, as well as prevention and treatment of alcohol abuse and dependence by pregnant women and by women at risk of becoming pregnant, should be a high, and long-term, priority of this coordinating body. Additional important areas of focus should include basic research and communication among the basic and clinical research communities and the health services community. Recommendations for research in all aspects of FAS can be found in this report and should serve as guidance for the coordinating body. Finally, the coordinating body should take active steps to encourage and facilitate the rigorous evaluation of all intervention programs.

Appendix

Biographies

FREDERICK C. BATTAGLIA (CHAIR) is Professor of Pediatrics, and Obstetrics-Gynecology, Division of Perinatal Medicine, University of Colorado Health Sciences Center. He received a B.A. degree from Cornell University and an M.D. from Yale University. He is a member of the Institute of Medicine. He has received the Agnes Higgins Award from the March of Dimes Birth Defects Foundation, the Nutrition Award and the Medical Education Award from the American Academy of Pediatrics. His research interests have centered around perinatal physiology as well as fetal and neonatal growth and nutrition. Dr. Battaglia is President-Elect of both the American Pediatric Society and the International Congress of Perinatal Medicine. He has served on the IOM committee on Fetal Research and Applications and on various committees for NIH and the March of Dimes Birth Defects Foundation.

HOOVER ADGER, JR. is Associate Professor in the Division of General Pediatrics and Adolescent Medicine, Johns Hopkins Hospital. He is a graduate of Ohio University and received an M.D. degree from Case Western Reserve University School of Medicine and an M.P.H. degree from the Johns Hopkins University School of Hygiene and Public Health. Dr. Adger completed residency training at the Children's Hospital Medical Center in Cincinnati and was awarded a fellowship in adolescent medicine at the University of California, San Francisco. He has served as president of the Association of Medical Education and Research in Substance Abuse.

NANCY C. ANDREASEN is Andrew H. Woods Professor of Psychiatry at the University of Iowa College of Medicine, and Director, Mental Health Clinical Research Center, University of Iowa Hospital and Clinics. She received B.A. and Ph.D. degrees from the University of Nebraska, an M.A. from Harvard University, and an M.D. degree from the University of Iowa. She was the recipient of a Fulbright Fellowship to Oxford University. She is a member of the Institute of Medicine. She is Editor-in Chief of the American Journal of Psychiatry and has served as President of the American Psychopathological Association and the Psychiatric Research Society. She is the recipient of the Research Prize of the American Psychiatric Association and the Dean Award and the Distinguished Service Award of the American College of Psychiatry. Dr. Andreasen also served on the American Psychiatric Association's task force for the Diagnostic and Statistical Manual of the Mental Disorders, Fourth Edition (DSM-IV) and chaired its Schizophrenia and Other Psychotic Disorders Work Group.

KATHLEEN M. CARROLL is Assistant Professor of Psychiatry and Director of Psychotherapy Research, Substance Abuse Center, Yale University School of Medicine. She received a B.S. degree from Duke University and M.A. and Ph.D. degrees in clinical psychology from the University of Minnesota. Dr. Carroll's research interests center around substance abuse treatment outcome research, including addicted women. She is a member of the American Psychological Association, the Society for Psychotherapy Research, and the Society for Psychologists in Addictive Behaviors. Dr. Carroll is a consulting editor for the journals *Psychological Assessment* and *Psychology of Addictive Behaviors*.

STERLING K. CLARREN is Robert A. Aldrich Professor of Pediatrics, Division of Congenital Defects, Children's Hospital and Medical Center, University of Washington. He is the director of the FAS Clinic at the Child Development and Mental Retardation Center, University of Washington and director of the State of Washington's FAS Clinical Network. He received a B.A. degree from Yale University and an M.D. degree from the University of Minnesota Medical School. At the University of Washington, Seattle, Dr. Clarren completed a pediatrics residency and received fellowships in biosciences, dysmorphology, and congenital defects. He has served as president of the Fetal Alcohol Syndrome Study Group of the Research Society on Alcoholism, on the Public Education Committee of the Teratology Society, and on the Executive Committee of the Children with Disabilities Section of the American Academy of Pediatrics. In 1992, he received the Outstanding Achievement Award for Scholarship from the Washington Council on Crime and Delinquency.

CLAIRE D. COLES is Associate Professor, Departments of Psychiatry and Pediatrics, Emory University School of Medicine. She also serves as Director of Psychological Services for the Marcus Developmental Research Center in the

Department of Pediatrics and as Director of Clinical and Developmental Research, Human and Behavioral Genetics Laboratory, in the Department of Psychiatry. Dr. Coles received a B.A. degree from Oglethorpe University and M.A. and Ph.D. degrees in developmental psychology from Emory University. She is a past president of the Fetal Alcohol Study Group of the Research Society on Alcoholism and serves on the executive committee of the Parent-Infant Resource Center of Georgia State University.

HENRY W. FOSTER, JR. is a practicing gynecologist and medical educator. Dr. Foster is Professor of Obstetrics and Gynecology at Meharry Medical College, where he had served as dean of the school of medicine and acting president, Dr. Foster recently has been scholar-in-residence at the Association of Academic Health Centers in Washington, D.C. Dr. Foster earned a B.S. degree from Morehouse College in 1954 and was awarded his M.D. degree by the University of Arkansas in 1958. He undertook an internship at the Detroit Receiving Hospital, served two years as a medical officer in the U.S. Air Force, and spent one year in residency training in general surgery at Malden Hospital in Massachusetts. He completed a three-year residency in obstetrics and gynecology at Meharry Medical College in Nashville. Dr. Foster is a member of the Institute of Medicine. He has received an Appreciation Award for Research and Teaching on Sickle Cell Anemia from Tuskegee University and a Faculty Award for Excellence in Science and Technology from the White House Initiative on Historically Black Colleges and Universities. He has served as an examiner for the American Board of Obstetrics and Gynecology and has been a member of the editorial board of the journal *Academia*.

DONALD E. HUTCHINGS is a Research Scientist at New York State Psychiatric Institute, Department of Developmental Psychobiology and in the Departments of Psychiatry and Pediatrics, Columbia College of Physicians and Surgeons. He received a B.A. from Lake Forest College and an M.A. and Ph. D. from the University of Chicago. His research includes preclinical studies of the developmental toxicity of substances of abuse as well as the addiction treatment compounds, methadone and buprenorphine. In addition to service on a committee of the National Research Council, Dr. Hutchings has served on review committees of the National Institute of Drug Abuse and advisory boards of the National Institute of Environmental Science and the National Institute of Occupational Safety and Health. He is a co-founder of the Neurobehavioral Teratology Society and Editor-in-Chief of *Neurotoxicology and Teratology*.

PHILIP A. MAY is Professor of Sociology and Psychiatry and Director of the Center on Alcoholism, Substance Abuse and Addictions at the University of New Mexico. He earned an A.B. degree from Catawba College, Salisbury, North Carolina, an M.A. from Wake Forest University, and a Ph.D. in sociology from the University of Montana. Dr. May's research has focused on the epidemiology and prevention of behavioral health problems: adult alcohol abuse, suicide, motor vehicle crashes, and for over fifteen years, FAS. He served on the U.S. Surgeon General's Workshop on Drunk Driving in 1988, and has received several awards, including a Certificate of Appreciation from the U.S. Bureau of Indian Affairs. Two special awards of recognition and appreciation have been presented to him from the U.S. Indian Health Service for Prevention of FAS among American Indians. More recently he was honored with a humanitarian award from the United Nations Association, New Mexico Chapter.

BENNETT A. SHAYWITZ is Professor of Pediatrics, Neurology and Child Study Center, and Chief of Pediatric Neurology at the Yale University School of Medicine. He is also Co-Director of the first federally funded Center for the Study of Learning and Attention Disorders. A graduate of Washington University (A.B., 1960; M.D., 1963), Dr. Shaywitz trained first in pediatrics and then child neurology at the Albert Einstein College of Medicine. Dr. Shaywitz's primary and long-standing research has focused on the neurobiological influences in learning and attention disorders. In addition to service on committees of the Institute of Medicine, Dr. Shaywitz has served on advisory boards and committees at the National Institutes of Health, and the Professional Advisory Board of the National Center for Children with Learning Disabilities.

ROBERT J. SOKOL is Dean of the School of Medicine and Professor in the Department of Obstetrics and Gynecology and Director of the Fetal Alcohol Research Center at Wayne State University. He also serves as Senior Vice President for Medical Affairs of the Board of the Detroit Medical Center. Dr. Sokol received B.A. and M.D. degrees from the University of Rochester (1963 and 1966). He completed a residency in obstetrics and gynecology at the Barnes Hospital/Washington University. He served in the U.S. Air Force from 1970 to 1972 after which he was awarded fellowships in maternal-fetal medicine at Strong Memorial Hospital in Rochester and at Cleveland Metropolitan Hospital. A past President of the Society of Perinatal Obstetricians, he recently received a Career Achievement Award from that organization. With a long-term goal to prevent perinatally incurred brain damage, Dr. Sokol's methodologic work focuses on Medical Informatics and Clinical Epidemiology. His current research addresses the neurobehavioral consequences of prenatal alcohol and drug exposure.

R. DALE WALKER is Professor, Department of Psychiatry and Behavioral Sciences, University of Washington School of Medicine. He is also Chief of the Addictions Treatment Center of the Veterans Affairs Medical Center in Seattle. Dr. Walker received B.S. and M.D. degrees from the University of Oklahoma and completed a residency in psychiatry at the University of California, San Diego. He was awarded a Fellowship in Public Health by the Andrija Stamper School of

Public Health in Zagreb, Yugoslavia, and a Fellowship in Gastroenterology by the Royal Free Hospital in London. He has served as secretary of the Association of American Indian Physicians, has chaired committees of the American Psychiatric Association, and was an invited participant at the U.S. Surgeon General's Workshop on Violence and Public Health in 1985. Dr. Walker received an Award for Outstanding Service from the Seattle Indian Health Board in 1985 and was named Physician of the Year by the Association of American Indian Physicians in 1989. Dr. Walker served on the Institute of Medicine committee that produced the report *Broadening the Base of Treatment for Alcohol Problems* in 1990.

JOANNE WEINBERG is Professor of Anatomy at the University of British Columbia in Vancouver. She received an A.B. degree from Brown University, an M.A.T. from Harvard, and a Ph.D. degree in neurosciences from Stanford University Medical School and undertook postdoctoral training in developmental psychobiology and in human nutrition. Dr. Weinberg is the current president of the Fetal Alcohol Syndrome Study Group and has served on the board of directors of the Research Society on Alcoholism and the International Society for Developmental Psychobiology. She is on the editorial advisory board of the journals *Physiology and Behavior*, *Alcohol*, and *Alcoholism: Clinical and Experimental Research*. Her research interests include fetal alcohol syndrome, psychosocial stressors and mouse mammary tumor growth, and the neurobiology of stress.

SHARON C. WILSNACK is Chester Fritz Distinguished Professor in the Department of Neuroscience and Director of Preclinical Curriculum in Psychiatry and Behavioral Science at the University of North Dakota School of Medicine. She received M.A. and Ph.D. degrees in clinical psychology from Harvard University and studied as a Fulbright Scholar at the University of Freiburg, Federal Republic of Germany. Dr. Wilsnack's background includes experience as an alcoholism therapist and treatment program director as well as in research and medical education. Her research interests include psychologic aspects of alcohol use and abuse in women, and longitudinal prediction of changes in drinking behavior. She is co-editor with Linda Beckman of the volume *Alcohol Problems in Women: Antecedents, Consequences, and Intervention* and is currently editing with Richard Wilsnack a book on gender and alcohol to be published by Rutgers University. Dr. Wilsnack served on the Institute of Medicine committee that produced the workshop summary *Assessing Future Research Needs: Mental and Addictive Disorders in Women* in 1991.

Institute of Medicine Staff

KATHLEEN R. STRATTON is a Senior Program Officer and the Associate Director of the Division of Health Promotion and Disease Prevention. She did undergraduate work in natural sciences at Johns Hopkins University, Baltimore, Maryland, and received her Ph.D. in pharmacology and toxicology from the University of Maryland at Baltimore. She did a post-doctoral research fellowship in the Department of Neuroscience at Johns Hopkins University School of Medicine. She has most recently finished a major project at the IOM on adverse consequences of childhood vaccines. Other projects during her six years at the National Research Council and the Institute of Medicine include work with the Committee to Study the Co-Administration of Research and Services at the National Institutes of Health and the Alcohol, Drug Abuse, and Mental Health Administration, Committee on Risk Assessment of Hazardous Air Pollutants, Committee on Risk Assessment Methodology and the Committee on Neurotoxicology and Models for Assessing Risks. Her next project concerns priorities for vaccine development.

CYNTHIA J. HOWE is a Program Officer in the Division of Health Promotion and Disease Prevention and the Division of Biobehavioral Sciences and Mental Disorders of the Institute of Medicine. She received a B.A. degree in psychology from Wittenberg University in Springfield, Ohio, and has done graduate work in experimental psychology at the University of Maryland, College Park. Other projects during 14 years at the Institute of Medicine include the Vaccine Safety Forum; studies of the adverse effects of childhood vaccines; and a study of chronic pain and disability. Ms. Howe, along with four colleagues, is a recipient of the National Research Council's 1992 Group Recognition Award, as well as the 1991 Group Achievement Award of the Institute of Medicine for her work on the report *Adverse Effects of Pertussis and Rubella Vaccines*.

DOROTHY R. MAJEWSKI is a Project Assistant in the Division of Health Promotion and Disease Prevention and the Division of Biobehavioral Sciences and Mental Disorders. She received a B.A. degree in education from Carlow College in Pittsburgh, Pennsylvania. During her seven years at the National Academy of Sciences she has worked on the current project on Fetal Alcohol Syndrome, as well as other projects on priorities for vaccine development, vaccine safety, adverse effects of childhood vaccines, and one on diet and health for the Food and Nutrition Board. Ms. Majewski, along with four colleagues, is a recipient of the National Research Council's 1992 Group Recognition Award, as well as the 1991 Group Achievement Award of the Institute of Medicine for her work on the report *Adverse Effects of Pertussis and Rubella Vaccines*.

Index

A

Aarskog syndrome, 79
Abstinence during pregnancy, 27, 103,
    105
  counseling for, 11, 146
  encouraged as means of FAS
    prevention, 9, 17, 27, 118
Academic performance, 69, 159, 163-164,
    165; *see also* Adolescence and post-
    puberty development
Acetaldehyde adducts, 129-130
Active surveillance, 7, 91, 94-96, 97
  linkages to treatment, 8, 97
  proxy measures, 7, 95-96
Adaptive functioning, 73, 159, 163
Adolescence and post-puberty
    development, 6, 36, 80, 158
  behavior patterns, 165-166, 168-169
  catch-up growth, 73, 75
Adoption, 13, 15, 67, 74, 171, 172, 181,
    186
Adulthood, 19, 75, 166
Affected individuals, *see* Behavioral
    patterns; Cognitive performance;
    Developmental stages and life span;

Diagnostic criteria; Growth
    deficiency; Incidence and
    prevalence of FAS; Physical
    anomalies; Secondary disabilities;
    Treatment and intervention for FAS
    children
African Americans
  FAS rates, 83
  maternal drinking patterns, 103
Age
  and drinking patterns, 106, 107, 108-
    109, 121
  and subsequent pregnancies, 136
  see also Developmental stages and life
    span
Aggression 163
Alanine aminotransferases (ALT), 128-
    129
Alcohol abuse, 117
  among FAS adolescents, 158
  biological markers, 9, 109, 126-131
  diagnostic definition, 5n, 29-30, 68,
    74, 77n
  social-environmental factors, 88-89,
    100-102, 108-109
  stigma of, 92, 94, 96, 112, 146

see also Drinking among women;
    Drinking during pregnancy; Heavy
    drinking; Treatment and prevention
    of alcohol abuse
Alcoholics Anonymous (AA), 140
Alcohol-related birth defects (ARBD), 3,
    5, 7, 77, 78-79, 80, 97
    incidence and prevalence, 84, 97
Alcohol-related effects (diagnostic
    category), 4-5, 76-77, 78-79, 80.
    see also "Fetal alcohol effects"
    diagnostic criteria, 4-5, 67, 70, 76-77,
    78
Alcohol-related neurodevelopmental
    disorder (ARND), 3, 5, 7, 77, 78-
    79, 80, 81, 97
    incidence and prevalence, 97
Alkaline phosphatase (AP), 129
Aminotransferases, 128-129
Anger, 80
Animal models and studies
    intervention and prevention strategies,
    11-12, 15, 45-47, 144, 147, 155,
    186
    paternal alcohol exposure, 121
    teratogenic effects, 6, 20, 22, 28, 37-
    41, 81
Antisocial behavior, 80
Anxiety, 80, 107, 108
Asian Americans, FAS rates, 83
Aspartate aminotransferases (AST), 128-
    129
Aspirin, 45-46
Attention, 15, 73, 159, 163, 164, 168, 186
Attention-deficit hyperactivity disorder
    (ADHD), 69, 161, 164, 177, 182
Autopsy studies, 72

B

Babies, see Newborn period and infancy
Bartenders, 122
Baseline data, 7, 89-90, 97
Behavioral patterns, 4, 5, 17, 43-44, 73,
    75, 76, 77, 81, 158-166
    across developmental stages, 69, 159-
    166, 168-169

as diagnostic criteria, 3, 67, 69
    etiology, 166-167, 169-173
    of FAS adolescents, 165-166, 168-169
    of newborns and infants, 160-161
    research needs, 15, 186
    research studies, 158-159
    specificity to FAS, 13, 79, 167, 173
    vignettes, 56-58
    see also Alcohol-related
    neurodevelopmental disorder
    (ARND)
Behavioral Risk Factors Surveillance
    Surveys (BRFSS), 100, 104, 105,
    106
Binge drinking, 44, 68, 106, 165, 166
Biological markers, 6, 72, 81, 115, 126-
    131, 135, 169
    of alcohol abuse, 9, 109, 126-131
    research needs, 6, 9, 81, 109
Birth, see Newborn period and infancy
Birth control, 11, 136, 146-147
Birth Defects Monitoring Program
    (BDMP), 22, 83, 91
Birth registries, 83, 84, 90
Birth to Three Project, 142
Blood alcohol levels, 127
Bloom syndrome, 79
Brain damage, 4, 38, 39-40, 44, 68, 71,
    72-73, 74, 75, 76, 81, 157, 169, 173
Brain stem auditory evoked response
    (BAER) test, 157
Breast-feeding, 142, 157
Breath analyzer, 127
Brief interventions, 10, 123-124, 131-135

C

CAGE test, 124, 126
Carbohydrate-deficient transferrin (CDT),
    130-131
Cardiac defects, 38, 156
Caregiving environment, 13, 53, 163, 165,
    169-173
Case management, 11, 142, 147
Categories, see Alcohol-related birth
    defects (ARBD); Alcohol-related
    neurodevelopmental disorder

(ARND); Diagnostic categories; FAS with confirmed maternal alcohol exposure; FAS without confirmed maternal alcohol exposure; Partial FAS

Caucasians/whites
  FAS rates, 83
  maternal drinking, 106, 107
Center for Substance Abuse Prevention (CSAP), 23
Center for Substance Abuse Treatment (CSAT), 23
Centers for Disease Control and Prevention (CDC)
  risk factor surveys, 100, 104, 105
  screening check lists, 72
  surveillance and prevention programs, 22, 28, 83-84, 91, 97, 136, 144-145, 176, 195
Central nervous system (CNS)
  dysfunction, 4, 33, 38, 39, 71, 75, 76, 91
Cerebellar hypoplasia, 69, 73
Child abuse, 53, 102, 142, 170, 173
Cigarettes, *see* Smoking
Clinical practice guidelines, 15, 186
Clinic-based studies, 8, 102, 103, 158
  FAS incidence and prevalence estimates, 83, 84-87
Cocaine, 21, 23, 36, 105, 137; *see also* Crack cocaine
Cognitive-behavioral interventions, 140
Cognitive performance, 4, 5, 17, 19, 73, 75, 76, 77, 81, 158, 159, 161, 163-164
  see also Alcohol-related neuro-developmental disorder (ARND); Mental retardation
Community involvement, 114-115, 122, 185
Computed tomography (CT), 69, 72
Confidentiality, 92, 141, 176, 186
Congenital rubella syndrome (CRS), 20-21
Contraceptive services, 11, 136, 146-147
Coordination of services, 15-16, 176, 183-184, 194-196
Coordination problems, 73

Corpus callosum
  callosal dysgenesis, 69, 73
Counseling
  for abstinence during pregnancy, 11, 146
  brief interventions, 10, 123-124, 131-135
  contraceptive services, 11, 136, 146-147
Crack cocaine, 21, 105, 137
Cranial size, 4, 68, 70, 76
Creatine phosphokinase (CPK), 127
Cross-sectional research, syndrome characteristics over life span, 80
Culture, *see* Ethnic groups; Social-environmental factors
Custody losses and retention, 11, 21, 142, 171-173; *see also* Foster care

D

Dental abnormalities, 156, 157
Depression, 80, 102, 107-108
Developmental delay, 6, 19, 73, 81, 135, 154, 161, 184
  research needs, 6, 81
Developmental stages and life span
  behavioral patterns across, 69, 159-166, 168-169
  diagnoses performed over, 6, 67, 70, 73-74, 80, 92
  interventions over, 15, 166, 167-169, 174-175, 186
  research needs, 6, 80, 167
  variability in outcomes, 13, 167-168
  worsening of effects over, 168-169
  see also Adolescence and post-puberty development; Adulthood; Newborn period and infancy; Preschool period; School age
Developmental toxicity, 33-37
Diagnoses and diagnostic labels
  consistency of, 64-65, 91-92
  history of FAS definition, 17-19, 70-73
  as marker for preventive interventions, 79-80
  problems in surveillance, 64, 84, 90, 91-92

and secondary disability prevention,
80, 182
uses of, 2, 63-64, 79-80
at various developmental stages, 6, 67,
70, 73-74, 80, 92
see also Biological markers
Diagnostic and Statistical Manual (DSM),
29-30, 64
Diagnostic categories, 3, 4-5, 74-79
Diagnostic criteria, 2-6, 64-70, 182, 185
for alcohol abuse and dependence, 5n,
29-30, 68, 74, 77n
alcohol-related effects, 4-5, 67, 70, 76-
77, 78
application across life span, 3, 6, 67,
70, 80
behavioral and cognitive features, 3,
67, 69
clinical applications, 64, 66, 67, 80
documented exposure to alcohol, 2, 3,
4, 6, 67-68, 74-75, 76, 80
physical features, 2, 67, 68
reliability and validity, 64-65, 71-72
research applications, 64, 66, 67, 80
research needs, 6, 80-81
role of imaging technology, 3, 67, 69,
69-70, 72-73
Dietary and nutrition factors, 9, 102, 109
fat intake, 46
Diethylbestrol (DES), 41
Differential diagnosis, 64, 79
Diphenylhydantoin (DPH, phenytoin), 34,
35, 41
Dose-response relationships, 41-45, 103,
112
Drinking among women, 9, 22, 100, 102,
105, 108, 109-110
heavy drinkers, 88, 105
low and moderate intake, 105
stigmatizing effects, 112, 146
Drinking contexts, 107
Drinking during pregnancy, 8-9, 103, 100-
107
bingeing, 44, 68, 106, 165, 166
documentation of, 2, 3, 4, 6, 67-68, 74-
75, 76, 80, 132

factors influencing, 9, 100-102, 106-
107, 109, 121, 147
fetal protection mechanisms, 9, 12,
109, 147
first trimester, 106-107
heavy drinking, 27, 89, 100-101, 106,
120, 121
low and moderate intake, 2, 26-27,
116, 117-118, 120
and multiple-substance use, 21, 109
as proxy indicator of FAS, 95-96, 143
reduction of intake, 105-106, 119-120,
133-134
research needs, 9, 107-110
variation among ethnic groups, 103,
108-109
vignettes, 53-62
see also Abstinence during pregnancy
Drugs, *see* Illicit drug use during
pregnancy
"Drunk" baby, 19
Dubowitz syndrome, 79
Dysmorphism, *see* Physical anomalies

E

Early intervention programs, 175, 176, 177
Eating disorders, 107
Education, *see* Academic performance;
Parenting education; Professional
training and education; Public
education campaigns
Educational interventions, 15, 186
for children with prenatal drug
exposure, 15, 186
for secondary disabilities, 14, 155,
174-175, 177-179
Eligibility for services, 155, 156, 182-183
Embryonic period, 38-39
Emotional health, 15, 173, 186
Environment, *see* Caregiving
environment; Social-environmental
factors
Epicanthal folds, 72
Epidemiology and surveillance, 6-7, 89-97
active surveillance, 7, 91, 94-96, 97

drinking among women, 9, 22, 100, 105, 108, 109-110

drinking during pregnancy, 8-9, 22, 100-109

FAS baseline data, 7, 89-90, 97

and FAS diagnostic problems, 64, 84, 90, 91-92

passive surveillance, 6-7, 83, 91-94

role in prevention programs assessment, 89-90, 97

use of multiple data sources, 84, 90-91

see also Clinic-based studies; Incidence and prevalence of FAS; Longitudinal studies; Population-based epidemiologic studies; Registry-based studies

Erythrocyte delta-aminolevulinic acid (ALA) dehydrase, 127-128

Ethnic groups

biomodal patterns of alcohol abuse, 88-89, 103

and maternal drinking, 103, 108-109, 121

variation in FAS prevalence estimates, 7, 90, 97

see also African Americans; Asian Americans, FAS rates; Caucasians/whites; Hispanics, FAS rates; Native Americans

Etiology, of behavioral patterns, 166-167, 169-173

Eyebrows, 72

Eye defects, 38, 72, 73, 157

F

Facial anomalies, 17, 38, 68, 70, 72, 73, 165

in diagnosis, 4, 73, 74, 75, 76

presence at birth, 71, 73, 160

Failure to thrive, 73, 157, 161

Families

alcohol abuse history in, 53, 102, 107

interventions and support, 11, 14, 14-15, 117, 142, 180-181, 185

involvement in mothers' alcohol reduction and cessation, 10, 11, 115, 122, 146, 147

stability of, 53, 170

see also Caregiving environment

FAS with confirmed maternal alcohol exposure (diagnostic category), 3, 4, 74, 76

FAS without confirmed maternal alcohol exposure (diagnostic category), 3, 4, 74-75, 76

Fathers, *see* Partners of women; Paternal alcohol exposure

"Fetal alcohol effects" (FAE), 3, 63, 67, 70, 78. *see also* Alcohol-related effects

Folic acid deficiency, 21

Follow-up in treatment, 15, 183, 186

Foster care, 11, 13, 74, 142, 171, 172, 181

Fragile-X syndrome, 69, 74, 79

G

Gamma glutamyl transferase (GGT), 128, 131

Gatekeeping, 66, 79, 182

Gender differences

alcohol treatment effectiveness, 139

biological markers for alcohol abuse, 128, 130-131

growth, 73

prenatal dose-response effects, 44

Genetic susceptibility, 40-41, 90

D-Glucaric acid, 127

Growth deficiency, 40, 71, 73-74, 157, 160

in diagnosis, 4, 70, 75, 76, 92, 160

low birthweight, 4, 40, 41, 68, 69-70, 76, 92-93

H

Head Start, 175, 177

Health care interventions, 12, 147, 176-177

brief interventions, 10, 123-124, 131-135

referrals, 10, 11, 15, 131-132, 135, 147, 184

screening for maternal alcohol use, 124-131

secondary disabilities, 174, 176-177
selective, 10, 123-133
training, 11, 15, 123, 132-133, 147, 184
universal, 118-119
Health Resources and Services
    Administration (HRSA), 23, 143,
    195
Healthy People 2000 goals, 20, 89-90
Hearing problems, 73, 157
Heavy drinking, 29, 30-31, 88, 105
definitions, 106
during pregnancy, 27, 89, 100-101,
    106, 120, 121
identification, 11, 123, 124-126, 132-
    133, 147
Heroin, 35
Hispanics, FAS rates, 83
Hospital discharge data, 83, 84, 91
Hydronephrosis, 156
Hyperactivity, 159, 160, 161, 163, 164, 182

I

Ibuprofen, 46
Illicit drug use during pregnancy, 21, 103,
    105, 109
educational interventions for children,
    15, 186
forced treatment and incarceration, 21,
    137
Imaging techniques, 45, 69, 71
role in establishing diagnostic criteria,
    3, 67, 69-70, 72-73
Impulse control, 164
Incarceration, of substance-abusing
    mothers, 21, 137
Incidence and prevalence of FAS
alternative estimates, 1, 6, 19, 27, 82-
    91
among ethnic minorities, 7, 83, 97
Income and socioeconomic status, 89,
    103, 106, 107, 108-109, 116-117,
    121, 155
Indian Health Service, 23, 144, 195
Indicated prevention interventions, 10, 11-
    12, 115, 135-141, 145-147

alcohol abuse treatment as, 9, 10, 11,
    107-108, 115, 135, 138-141, 141,
    145, 154
for mothers of FAS children, 79, 135,
    136-137
reproductive counseling and
    contraceptive services, 11, 136,
    146-147
research needs, 11-12, 146-147
Indomethacin, 46
Infants, see Newborn period and infancy
Integration and coordination of services,
    15-16, 176, 183-184, 194-196
Intellect, see Cognitive performance
Interagency cooperation, 15-16, 195-196
national survey, 7, 16, 97, 196
task force, 16, 196
Intervention, see Educational
    interventions; Health care
    interventions; Prevention
    interventions and measures;
    Treatment and intervention for FAS
    children; Treatment and prevention
    of alcohol abuse
IQ scores, 159, 163
Iron deficiency anemia, 131
Isolation, 80
Isotreinoin, 42

J

Judgment, 73, 158, 163

K

Kidney anomalies, 156

L

Labeling, see Diagnoses and diagnostic
    labels; Warning labels
Language development and deficits, 15,
    73, 159, 161-163, 186
Lead, 34, 35
Learning disabilities, 73

Liver damage, 127
Longitudinal studies, 19, 80, 86-87, 167
Low and moderate drinking, 105
    during pregnancy, 2, 26-27, 116, 117-
    118, 120
Low birthweight, 4, 40, 41, 68, 69-70, 76,
    92-93

M

Magnetic resonance imaging (MRI), 45,
    69, 71
Maintenance and aftercare, 114, 142
Males, *see* Gender differences; Partners of
    women
Mandatory drug testing, 21
March of Dimes, 133
Marijuana, 34, 36, 42
Marital status, 107, 121, 122
Maternal and Child Health Bureau
    (MCHB), 23, 143
Maternal Health Practices and Child
    Development (MHPCD) Project,
    93, 102
Maternal mortality, 171
Maternal PKU, 79
Math ability, 73, 159, 163-164, 166, 168
Mean corpuscular volume (MCV), 129
Media campaigns, 116, 147
Medical interventions, *see* Health care
    interventions
Medical records, 84, 90, 92, 94
Memory, 163
Mental retardation, 19, 159, 169, 173
    FAS as leading nongenetic cause, 7, 97
Methadone, 35
Methylmercury, 34, 35
Methylphenidate, 177
Metropolitan Atlanta Congenital Defects
    Program (MACDP), 83-84
Michigan Alcoholism Screening Test
    (MAST), 126
Microcephaly, 69, 72, 92
Middle class populations, 89, 103, 155
Minorities, *see* Ethnic groups
Moderate drinking, *see* Low and moderate
    drinking

Motivational interviewing, 140
Multidisciplinary approaches to service,
    15, 16, 194-196
Muscle tone, 73

N

National Fetal Mortality Survey, 104
National Health and Nutrition
    Examination Survey, 104
National Institute on Alcohol Abuse and
    Alcoholism (NIAAA), 16, 21-22,
    28, 144, 195, 196
National Institute on Drug Abuse (NIDA),
    21, 22
    pregnancy survey, 104, 105
National Institutes of Health (NIH), 21-22
National Longitudinal Alcohol
    Epidemiologic Study, 104
National Longitudinal Survey of Youth
    (NLSY), 104, 105
National Maternal and Infant Health
    Interview Survey (NMIHS), 104,
    105, 106
National Natality Survey, 104
National Organization on Fetal Alcohol
    Syndrome (NOFAS), 133
National Pregnancy and Health Survey,
    22, 104, 105
National surveys, 7, 97, 108, 109
    on drinking and pregnancy, 9, 102-
    103, 104, 108, 109
    interagency cooperation in, 7, 16, 97,
    196
Native Americans
    incarceration of pregnant women, 137
    maternal drinking patterns, 88-89, 103
    substance abuse treatment programs, 23
    surveillance, 83, 87-89, 93
Neglect, 53, 142, 157, 170, 171, 173
Neonatal withdrawal syndrome, 135, 160
Neural tube defects, 21
Neurobehavioral deficits, *see* Behavioral
    patterns
Neurobiological indicators, *see* Biological
    markers
Neurotoxicity, 33-36, 38, 39-40, 157

Newborn period and infancy
   associated health conditions, 156
   behavior patterns, 160-161
   blood alcohol levels, 19
   diagnosis during, 19, 70, 75, 91, 93-94,
     168
   environment enrichment, 46
   low birthweight, 4, 40, 41, 68, 69-70,
     76, 92-93
Non-steroidal anti-inflammatory (NSAI)
   agents, 46
Noonan's syndrome, 79
Normative standards, 68, 69

O

Obstetrician gynecologists, 118-119, 124,
   133, 194
Occupational therapy, 176, 177
Ocular problems, *see* Eye defects
Opiates, 34, 35-36
Opitz syndrome, 79
Organogenesis, 38
Otitis media, 157, 161
Outcomes research, alcohol treatment for
   women, 138-141

P

Palpebral fissures, 4, 72, 76
Parenting education, 15, 180-181, 185
Parity, 47, 136
Partial FAS (diagnostic category), 3, 4,
   75, 76, 78
Partners of women
   drinking behavior, 102, 107, 108, 121
   stability of relations with, 53, 107, 122
   targeted for interventions, 10, 11, 117,
     121-122, 142, 146
Passive surveillance, 6-7, 83, 91-94, *see*
   also Registry-based studies
   direct measures, 92
   indirect measures, 92-94
Paternal alcohol exposure, 121-122
Pattern recognition, 72
Pediatric specialties, 176, 194

Peers and friendships, 163
   of pregnant women, 10, 122
Perinatal 20 demonstration project, 22
Phenylketonuria, 79
Physical anomalies, 17-19, 156-157, 159
   as diagnostic criteria, 2, 67, 68
   prenatal development, 37-40
   see also Alcohol-related birth defects
     (ARBD); Facial anomalies; Growth
     deficiency
Physical therapy, 176, 177
Physician involvement, *see* Health care
   interventions
Placental growth, 69, 70
Polychlorinated biphenyls (PCBs), 34,
   35
Population-based epidemiologic studies,
   7, 87-89, 96
   drinking during pregnancy, 83, 95,
     102-103
Poverty areas and inner cities, 89, 103,
   155
Prader-Willi syndrome, 74
Predifferentiation period, 37-38
Pregnancy, *see* Abstinence during
   pregnancy; Drinking during
   pregnancy
Pregnancy Risk Assessment Monitoring
   System (PRAMS), 106
Pregnant and Postpartum Women and
   Their Infants (PPWI) initiative, 23,
   142-143
Prenatal care, 107, 124, 126-127, 133-135
Prenatal development, susceptibility over,
   36, 37-40
Preschool period
   behavior patterns, 161-163, 168
   services, 174, 177, 183
Prevalence, *see* Incidence and prevalence
   of FAS
Prevention interventions and measures, 9-
   12, 112-113
   birth defects, 20-21
   case management approaches, 114,
     142, 147
   comparison among programs, 11, 146

evaluation of impacts, 11, 16, 113, 119-120, 142-144, 146, 147, 196
indicated, 10, 11-12, 115, 135-141, 145-147
models of, 113-114
research needs, 11-12, 113, 146-147
research programs, 22-23, 144-145
secondary disabilities, 13-15, 80, 154, 173-181, 182-183, 185-186, 196
selective, 9-10, 12, 115, 120-135, 145, 147
universal, 9, 12, 114-115, 116-120, 145, 147
Problem solving, 163
Professional training and education
diagnosis of FAS, 66, 91, 92, 94, 133, 182
identification of heavy drinking, 11, 123, 132-133, 147
in prevention of FAS, 15, 132-133, 136, 179-180, 185
referral for treatment, 11, 15, 147, 184
Prospective studies, 83, 84, 86-87, 158-159
on effects of maternal substance use, 7, 26-27, 93, 94
Prostaglandin (PG), 45-46
Protective factors
against fetal injury, 9, 12, 45-46, 109, 147
women's drinking reduction, 9, 109, 147
Proxy indicators
of prevention activities impacts, 119, 143-144
surveillance criteria, 7, 92-94, 95-96
validation, 96
Psychological factors, 9, 102, 107, 109, 147
Psychotherapeutic drugs, 105, 177
Ptosis, 72
Puberty, *see also* Adolescence and post-puberty development
Public education campaigns, 9, 20, 116
Public Health Service (USPHS), 19, 20, 21-23

R

Racial groups, *see* Ethnic groups
Radiation, 34, 35
Referrals, 10, 11, 15, 131-132, 135, 147, 184
professional training in, 11, 15, 147, 184
Registry-based studies, 7, 83-84
Research needs
alcohol abuse, 9, 27-28, 102, 107-110, 138, 139, 141
behavioral patterns, 15, 186
biological markers, 6, 9, 81, 109
developmental stages, 6, 80, 167
diagnostic criteria, 6, 80-81
prevention interventions, 11-12, 113, 146-147
Research programs and studies, 21-23, 144-145
behavioral patterns, 158-159
coordination of, 15-16, 107, 194-196
prevention interventions, 22-23, 144-145
teratogenic effects, 19-20, 27, 37-45, 158
see also Animal models and studies; Clinic-based studies; Cross-sectional research; Epidemiology and surveillance; Longitudinal studies; National surveys; Population-based epidemiologic studies; Prospective studies; Research needs
Residential Treatment for Women and Their children, 23
Retrospective studies, 83, 84, 86, 158
Risk factors, *see* Dietary and nutrition factors; Social-environmental factors
Rubella, 20-21

S

Salicylate, 42
School age, 163-165, 168, 183

School performance, *see* Academic performance
Screening tools, 11, 146; *see also* Biological markers
Secondary disabilities, 12, 13-14, 80, 154-155, 173-181
  and caregiving environment, 155, 169-173
  educational interventions, 14, 155, 174-175, 177-179
  medical interventions, 174, 176-177
Seizures, 73, 157-158
Selective prevention interventions, 9-10, 12, 115, 120-135, 145, 147
  biological markers, 126-131
  brief interventions, 123-124, 131-135
  health care professionals' roles, 10, 123-133
  and prenatal care, 133-135
  professional training, 132-133
  referrals, 131-132
  research needs, 12, 147
  screening instruments, 124-126
  targeting of demographic subgroups, 12, 147
  targeting of family, 115, 122, 147
  targeting of women's partners, 121-122
Self-esteem, 102, 107, 140
Self-help groups, 140
Sensory integration, 15, 161, 163, 186
Skeletal anomalies, 38, 156
Sleep disturbances, 160
Smoking, 34, 36, 101, 105, 121
Social-environmental factors, 9, 90, 109, 147
  in alcohol abuse, 88-89, 100-102, 108-109
  role in modifying fetal alcohol exposure, 15, 46-47, 186
Socioeconomic status, *see* Income and socioeconomic status
Species susceptibility, 40
Speech delays, 73, 157
Stability of relationships, 53, 107, 121, 171-173
State-based surveys, 22, 97

State government agencies, 195
Stigma
  of alcohol abuse, 92, 94, 96, 112, 146
  of FAS diagnosis, 2, 66
Substance Abuse and Mental Health Services Administration (SAMHSA), 23, 143, 195
Support groups, 140, 181
Surgeon General's warning, 2, 22, 27, 118
Surveillance, *see* Epidemiology and surveillance
Sweden, FAS rate, 84

T

T-ACE test, 125, 126
Targeting, *see* Indicated prevention interventions; Selective prevention interventions
Teratogenic effects, 33-36, 73, 101, 121, 159-160
  dose-response effects, 41-45
  low-level alcohol use, 27
  multifactorial model, 47-48
  research studies, 19-20, 27, 37-45, 158
Thalidomide, 41, 42
Therapeutic intervention, 176-177
Tobacco, *see* Smoking
Training, *see* Professional training and education
Treatment and intervention for FAS children, 12-14, 27-28, 173-186
  availability of services, 156, 175-176
  barriers to services, 155-156, 175-176, 181-184
  community outreach programs, 185
  coordination of services, 15, 16, 195, 196
  early identification, 14, 80, 155, 168, 182, 185
  eligibility for services, 155, 156, 182-183
  follow-up, 15, 183, 186
  local and regional clusters, 14, 185
  planning, 166-173

Treatment and prevention of alcohol abuse
   availability of services, 10-11, 137, 138, 141
   in drug treatment programs, 21
   evaluation of effectiveness, 138-141, 143-144
   forced, 21, 137
   intensive, 10-11, 140-141, 146
   as a preventive intervention for FAS, 9, 10, 107-108, 115, 135, 138, 145, 154
   referrals, 10, 135
   research needs and barriers, 27-28, 102, 138, 139, 141
Tremors, 73
Turner's syndrome, 79
TWEAK test, 125, 126
Twin studies, 41, 121

U

Universal prevention interventions, 9, 12, 114-115, 116-120, 145, 147
   health care professionals' roles, 118-119
   research needs, 12, 147

Urinary dolichol, 127-128
Urine testing, 21, 127-128
Urogenital problems, 38, 156

V

Velocardiofacial syndrome, 79
Vigilance, 164
Violence against women, 102, 107, 108
Vision problems, 73, 156, 157
Vitamin A, 42

W

Warning labels, 118, 119-120
Whites, *see* Caucasians/whites
Wiedemann-Beckwith syndrome, 74
Williams syndrome, 79
Women's drinking, *see* Drinking among women; Drinking during pregnancy